Your Prostate Answer Book

Natural Remedies
vs.
Medical Options

and What Your Doctor
May Not Know

Publisher's Note

"I am the vine; you are the branches. If a man remains in me and I in him, he will bear much fruit; apart from me you can do nothing."

John 15:5 (NLT)

FC&A Medical Publishing®
103 Clover Green
Peachtree City, GA 30269

Produced by the staff of FC&A

ISBN 978-1-935574-16-3

Table of contents

Don't miss this introduction 1

Part 1 — You and your prostate

1 The prostate and the PSA: what men must know NOW . . . 10

The PSA test is "a hugely expensive public health disaster." And that warning comes from the man who discovered the PSA, a test that has led to the overdiagnosis and overtreatment of prostate cancer in hundreds of thousands of men.

2 PSA: knowing the real score 19

The PSA is far from perfect as a screening test for prostate cancer. It can indicate cancer when there is none and miss life-threatening disease. However, these are not the reasons why many experts believe the test should be shelved and dismissed as a medical mistake. Here's everything you need to know about whether to test — or not.

Benefits, limitations, and uncertainties 20
Where's the informed consent that's truly informed? 22
Need-to-know information 24
What to do after your PSA test 28
The two sides to this story 30

Part 2 — When things go wrong

3 What can go wrong: common prostate problems 34

In life, the saying goes, two things are certain — taxes and death. In a man's life you could add another — prostate trouble. Ninety percent of men will experience some type of prostate problem in their lifetime, largely due to the unusual anatomy and habitat of the prostate gland. Here's what can go wrong — and what you can do about it.

Benign prostatic hyperplasia: your growing prostate. 38
Prostatitis: when infection sets in 70
Prostate stones: blocked ducts 86

4 When the doctor says it's cancer. 87

Though there is nothing good about a diagnosis of cancer, there is some good news when the diagnosis is prostate cancer. The majority of men diagnosed with prostate cancer have early-stage disease, meaning it's quite possible that it may never be a threat to you in your lifetime.

Why me?. 89
Testosterone: fueling cancer 91
How prostate cancer spreads 92
Signs and symptoms. 93
Is biopsy for you? 95
What to expect when you are expecting a biopsy 96
Consider the results. 98
Biopsy is not risk-free 98
Three kinds of cancer 99
How tumor grade is determined 102
Tests and more tests 104
Ask the crucial questions. 106

5 Prostate cancer: the wise man's guide to making the right decision 107

It's unfathomable to hear the diagnosis of cancer and not think about treating it. Most people — and this includes many doctors — are of a mind that cancer is so ominous that it must be caught early and treated aggressively to avoid what would otherwise be a painful and premature death. This is turning out not to be the case.

Active surveillance: watch and wait. 111
Surgery: out with the prostate. 115
Radical prostatectomy: popular by 'demand'. 120
Nerve-sparing prostatectomy: the big gamble. 122
Laparoscopic radical prostatectomy: the 'minimalist' 124
Robotic prostatectomy: hands-off surgery 126
External beam radiation: zap therapy. 130
Proton beam radiation: the nuclear reaction 133
Brachytherapy: highest cure rate, least side effects. 135

Androgen deprivation therapy: putting cancer in remission 140
Surgical castration: the path of most resistance 148
Cryoablation surgery: freeze therapy 149
High-intensity focused ultrasound: heat therapy 151
Comparing treatments 154

6 Assuring the best treatment for you: how to work with your doctor 170

Men make lousy patients. This is not just a casual observation. It's in your best interest — and your quality of life — to speak up. Know what to say and what to ask so you do what is best for you.

The most inconvenient truth 171
Help your urologist help you 173
Just routine procedure — or is it? 175
Why you want a second opinion 178
Find out about all your options 180
15 questions to ask a surgeon. 180

7 Quality of life issue: getting help for incontinence 182

Incontinence isn't life-threatening, but it is life-altering. For many men it is devastating. It can have such a profound effect on men who undergo prostate surgery that it leaves many of them feeling hopeless. It shouldn't. There are helpful solutions to this problem.

Why incontinence is a risk. 183
4 kinds of incontinence 184
Surgery and incontinence 186
Start with small artillery. 187
Bringing out the brigade 191
A word on proctitis 193

8 Rekindling your love life: a sex survival guide. 195

Though a prostate problem can sometimes make lovemaking difficult, it does not cause impotence. The treatments for prostate diseases cause impotence.

The mechanics of an erection set 196
From trauma to traumatic 197
Consider your state of stress. 198

Back in the saddle again 202
Oral medication: vitamin V for victory 203
Vasodilators: erection by injection 206
Vacuum pump: inflation at its best 208
Surgery: the main squeeze 209

Part 3 — The prostate protection plan

9 The prostate-protecting lifestyle: live like an ancient Greek . . 212

In very many ways, prostate disease is a "lifestyle disease," created by the Western style of living. Evidence shows that when men, who live in countries where the rate of prostate disease is low, adopt the Western lifestyle, they also adopt Western man's high risk of prostate disease.

Back to the 60s: the retro-Grecian formula 214
Secrets of the Mediterranean 215
How to avoid prostate surgery 216
The prostate-protecting lifestyle 218
Eat like an ancient Greek 219
Remember, what's good for the heart is good for the prostate 220
Watch your weight — go down 221
Watch your waist — get leaner 223
Get a move on 225
Find the path of most resistance 226
Get a special perk from a physically intense job 226
Salut! Make a toast to the prostate 227
Don't burn the midnight oil 228
Relax while changing your diet 230
Snuff the cigarettes and cigars 231
Monogamous sex is the only true 'safe sex' 232

10 Foods that promote prostate health 233

One of the most enjoyable ways you can pamper your prostate is to feed it well. Here's smart advice on a diet designed to keep your prostate healthy and treat it when it's sick. Get your fill of the foods that target prostate health.

Alliums: garlic and onions head the 'A' team 242

Apples: one a day keeps the oncologist away 246
Berries: fighting cancer by the spoonful 246
Cabbages: meet the crucifer clan. 247
Chilies: a hot choice to put the brakes on aggressive cancer 249
Citrus fruit: the best vitamin C solution 251
Cranberries: equal opportunity infection protection. 252
Fish: chewing the omega-3 fat. 253
Grapes: prostate benefits in a bunch 257
Green tea: the terminator. 258
Licorice: candy for the prostate 259
Mustard and mustard seeds: a healthy topping. 260
Olive oil: pouring with good health 261
Pomegranate juice and seeds: mega-trendy protection. 263
Pumpkin seeds: relief from the symptoms of BPH 265
Raisins: more than a trace of protection 267
Rosemary: keep it by the grill 268
Soy: thumbs up for Asian style 269
Spinach: the king of greens 271
Tomatoes: now we're cookin'! 273
Walnuts: snacking on vitamin E. 276
Whole grains: hearty options for a healthy prostate 277

11 Supplemental insurance: nutritional protection 281

*Researchers are investigating many substances — including
phytonutrients, herbs, and vitamins — with promising potential
to prevent and treat prostate disease. It's possible one could
someday help lead to a cure.*

First, some caveats 282
Aspirin: thinning your cancer risk 284
Vitamin D: don't forget the sunshine vitamin. 285
Quercetin: fighting prostate pain 287
Green tea extract: getting EGCG the easy way 289
Curcumin: India's gift to prostate health 290
African plum extract: a capsule a day helps keep BPH away 292
Lycopene: the prostate's little helper 293
Resveratrol: wine in a capsule 296
Fish oil: striving for balance. 297
Pectin: modified to fight cancer. 300
Grape seed extract: a wine alternative 301
Beta-sitosterol: helps with urinary control 302
Black cumin: the seed of good health 303

Lupeol: medicinal mango. 305
Black cohosh: relief for symptoms of advanced disease 306
Vitamin E: protective oil. 307
Zinc: an aphrodisiac for prostate health. 308
Beta carotene: not the final word. 310
Vitamin C: cast in controversy. 311
Conjugated linoleic acid: a good fat for the prostate 312
Selenium: protection — for some? 314
Aged garlic extract: concentrated prostate protection?. 316
Ellagic acid: support for chemotherapy 316
Red clover: an experimental herb of interest 318
Genistein: more than a hill of beans 319
Rye grass pollen extract: sleep better at night. 320
Fisetin: a possible healer on the horizon? 321
Bee pollen extract: a honey of a symptom fighter 322
Capsaicin: hot on the cancer trail. 323
Flaxseed oil: the fish oil alternative 324
Hops: brewing a secret nutrient. 326
Saw palmetto: prostate protection, Southern style 327
Stinging nettle extract: the 'hurt' that heals 330

Part 4 — Resources

12 Support groups: why they matter 332

13 America's top treatment centers for prostate disease 342

14 Prostate terminology defined. 347

Index 363

Don't miss this introduction

Let's make a deal!

Let's talk man to man. Pretend I'm a urologist and I just diagnosed you with early-stage prostate cancer. This means you have cancer in the small gland that makes the protective and lubricating fluid your body expels with semen during ejaculation. I tell you I want to cut out your prostate gland because that's your best choice for getting rid of the cancer. If you do nothing, I say, the cancer will get worse. Every day counts.

But, I frankly tell you that there's no guarantee the operation will be completely successful because the cancer may have spread. Nevertheless, having the operation may increase your chance of survival. Sounds like a no-brainer decision. Right?

But wait! There's a catch!

There are a few "little problems" the urologist in this scenario glossed over. You'll have to give up something in return for having the surgery. You won't have much bladder control, so you'll have to wear a diaper. Oh, and kiss your love life goodbye. Incontinence and impotence are part of the package, at least for a few weeks or months, and possibly much longer. One or both of these problems is more likely than not to plague you to some degree for the rest of your life.

You have to understand, prostate surgery is delicate and difficult. There's no room for error. Heck, even the best surgeons in the world can't promise a guy that complete urinary and sexual function will return. This is the bottom line for most prostate removal surgeries.

There are no guarantees. The dubious benefit of perhaps a small increase in life expectancy — of about six months on average — is all you may get in exchange for major, life-changing side effects that last for a lifetime in many men. Now, isn't that a great deal!

Think you might take a pass on the surgeon's offer to cut out your prostate gland? If so, you are in a very small minority. This surgery, called radical prostatectomy, and all the side effects that go with it is, by far, the most common choice in America for dealing with prostate cancer. And here's another reality, incredible but true: Radical prosta-tectomy is the treatment recommended by surgeons and accepted by 90 percent of men with early-stage, low-risk prostate cancer — a disease that may never be a life-threatening issue for them in their life-time. The great majority of men with early-stage prostate cancer most likely will wind up dying of something other than that disease.

Why?

Because prostate cancer is different than other cancers. It grows slowly, so slowly, in fact, that many times more men die with prostate cancer than die from prostate cancer. This cancer is usually nonthreatening and very common. It usually grows so slowly that most elderly men who die from other causes are found to have undetected prostate cancer when there is a thorough autopsy of the gland!

So why are so many men taking such a big gamble with their quality of life and opting for the most aggressive treatment when there are better options in most cases? Men aren't favoring surgery because they're stupid, but because they are scared. And naive. The way our medical system has been dealing with prostate cancer is a travesty beyond comprehension. Men are opting for surgery because urolo-gists aren't being square with them about all the facts involving prostate cancer — including alternative treatments that are proven to be better and safer in most cases.

Chief among the better treatments that don't require radical surgery is using a needle to implant in the prostate tiny radioactive seeds that can kill the cancer and then stop giving off radiation. This much less invasive procedure is called brachytherapy. It is proving to have a better cure rate than surgery and rarely causes incontinence or impotence. Better yet, after a diagnosis of early-stage prostate cancer is the option of doing nothing at all except keeping tabs on the dis-ease with regular checkups until — or if ever — treatment is needed.

However, instead of counseling their patients about active surveillance, as this "let's wait and see if the cancer becomes threatening" option is called, urologists usually recommend what they do best and, forgive my bluntness, what brings in the most money — radical surgery.

Now, the cat's out of the bag! As you'll discover in this book, the medical community is well aware that hundreds of thousands of men unnecessarily have had their prostates, and quality of life, surgically removed. It's also apparent that doctors are being too slow to do anything about the overuse of surgery. What's going on, or should we say, what's gone wrong with prostate cancer treatment in America may be an open secret among physicians, but the word isn't streaming down to those who have the most to lose — the men radically affected by often unnecessary surgery.

Every day in the United States, a typical scenario is being played out, just like this true-life one that took place with an acquaintance of ours who lives near Philadelphia, Pa.

Rick's story

Rick had regular prostate-specific antigen (PSA) tests as part of his annual physical exam. After Rick's PSA jumped from a 2 to a 4, his family doctor sent him to a urologist, who ordered a biopsy. The biopsy uncovered prostate cancer localized to the right side of the prostate gland.

Rick thoroughly researched the prognosis for his cancer before talking to his urologist about treatment options. Rick knew that his cancer was early-stage and that there were many options that might be better than rushing into surgery.

Rick recalls the conversation when he met with his urologist to discuss the biopsy results.

Urologist: "You need to have your prostate removed. It's fairly routine surgery; I do it every day. I've done thousands of these surgeries."

Rick: "Well, what does the cancer mean? What's my prognosis?"

Urologist: "If you have surgery, we'll get the cancer out and you'll be done with it. No radiation, no chemotherapy." (No mention that radiation, either by external beam or seed implant, is an alternative to surgery, or that chemotherapy is only used as a last resort for prostate cancer that has already spread.)

Rick: "What about side effects?" (Though he already knew what they were.)

Urologist: "I'll be honest, you'll have incontinence for a while and you'll have to wear adult diapers, but it'll just be for a few weeks." (Studies show that incontinence can last up to a year and uncontrollable leakage, called stress incontinence, commonly lasts a lifetime.)

Rick: "Wh-wh-at about my sex life?"

Urologist: "Well, we can do nerve-sparing surgery to save the nerves so you can still get an erection. It's what I'll try to do, but I can make no promises." (No mention that even with nerve-sparing surgery, it would be a long haul before Rick could resume his love life and, if and when it did come back, he'd likely need a frequent assist from expensive medicine like Viagra and Cialis.)

Rick: "When would I need to have this done?" (It was two days before Christmas.)

Urologist: "As soon as possible. I recommend you schedule surgery today before you leave the office. This is an aggressive disease and you can't wait." (Not true on both counts.)

Rick: "What about brachytherapy — seed implants?" (He had heard about the procedure but didn't know much about it.)

Urologist: "Well, I don't do them, so I can't recommend them either way. Not every man is a candidate for seeds." (Though other doctors in his practice did do seed implants, which he didn't mention.)

Rick: "Well, am I a candidate for seed implants?"

Urologist: "You're borderline, I'd say. And it may not work." (He's thinking but does not say, And if it doesn't work you'll sue me.)

Rick: "Well, I need to think about this. Can I get back to you?" (He just wants to get out of the office.)

Urologist: "Well, I wouldn't wait. My surgical schedule gets very full. You should schedule surgery now, because time is of the utmost. You can always cancel. You just don't want to wait too long. This disease is a killer and I can tell you that if you do nothing, you will die." (With these exaggerations, he could have added, and have a Merry Christmas!)

So with conversations like that going on in doctors' offices, you can see why so many men end up with a radical prostatectomy and its aftermath.

It's American tradition to trust your doctor. It's also impossible to think of cancer and not want to take it out. Surgical removal of most cancers, if possible, is generally the best treatment. But prostate cancer is different because it is usually so slow-growing that it doesn't progress to become life-threatening. Men are acting out of fear of cancer and ignorance that there are generally other and better alternatives.

Now, let's imagine another scenario that might have happened with a better doctor.

Rick's story II: what might have been

Urologist: "Well, I'm sorry to say that your biopsy shows you have cancer, but the news is good. The pathology report shows it's early-stage cancer, meaning it is low-risk."

Patient: "Cancer! Oh, no! This is terrible. I can't believe it! What will I do?" (He doesn't yet comprehend the words low-risk.)

Urologist: "Well, there are several treatment options, which I will thoroughly explain to you. But there's another option, as well — no treatment. It's called active surveillance. It means you'll have to have a physical and your PSA tested in three months and, if nothing is changed, every six months after that. This cancer usually grows at a snail's pace. It can take decades before it becomes dangerous. If we get to the point where it shows the cancer is progressing, then it's time to consider treatment."

Patient: "Gee, well I don't know. Sounds a little risky."

Urologist: "Not if you have all your tests and checkups like you're supposed to. There's no missing them! Being on active surveillance means you'll have to have another biopsy at some point and maybe even several to monitor the disease. You'll have to do this for the rest of your life." (You're not getting off scot-free, you know.)

Patient: "How safe is it?" (Sounds skeptical.)

Urologist: "Studies have proven that it's a safe alternative for a man with this early-stage disease profile. There is plenty of evidence showing that there is generally no better outcome for men with early-stage prostate cancer who rush into surgery than for men who wait months or years to get treated. In fact, studies show men who opt for active surveillance of prostate cancer that's not advanced have no greater risk of dying from prostate cancer than men who rush into surgery."

Patient: "So you mean I just do nothing now but get another PSA test and come back to see you in three months?" (He's starting to calm down.)

Urologist: "Well, not exactly. You could take better care of yourself. Studies show that you can reduce your odds of the cancer advancing — in fact, men can help prevent prostate cancer — by making healthy lifestyle changes. Walk a little more each day. Eat more fruits and veggies and less fat and sugar. Make sure you eat the right nutrients." (There are even studies showing that taking a daily aspirin may eventually prove to be very helpful in preventing the progression and spread of prostate cancer.)

Patient: "I didn't know that! How much can it really help?" (He sounds doubtful.)

Urologist: "It's estimated that as much as 90 percent of aggressive cases of this cancer could be avoided if American men followed better health habits. In fact, there are a lot of positive lifestyle changes you can make to help protect your prostate. I think you'll find them appealing. I'll give you a brochure that tells you all about it before you leave."

Patient: "So what should I do? What do you recommend? I mean, I've got cancer. This is much too great a decision to make on my own."

Urologist: "I can't make the decision for you. Ultimately, it is something you'll have to decide on your own. But I can help you. Let's sit down and I'll explain all the treatment options available to you. Then, you should take time to think about it. Talk it over with your wife and others in your life who you trust. I'll give you information to take with you on all the treatments we're discussing so you can review them with your loved ones. Please feel free to call me if you have any questions. We can discuss this more in a few weeks when you're ready. There is no rush."

Patient: "But, it's cancer! What do you mean by no rush?"

Urologist: "Prostate cancer is unlike other cancers. It grows very slowly. You won't gain a thing by making a decision today. You've just learned you have cancer. You're understandably emotional and you don't want to make an emotional decision. Just call me if you need me. If you'd like, you should get a second opinion."

Now, if this were the kind of conversation most men have with their doctors, do you think 90 percent of them would say, "Well, what the heck. Let's do surgery. You could use the money. Besides, my love life just ain't what it used to be anyway. Diapers? So what's the big deal!"

Hardly. There is no logical explanation why men who don't need surgery, and possibly never will need surgery, are willingly having it. The only possible explanation is that there is something broken in the system. Men aren't getting the straight facts about prostate cancer and all treatment options. An epidemic of unnecessary surgeries has occurred since widespread use of the PSA test started nearly 20 years ago. The doctor who discovered prostate-specific antigen (PSA), leading to the development of the PSA test, now says that use of this test is responsible for the overdiagnosis and overtreatment of prostate cancer.

Unfortunately, it's the exceptional surgeon who balances the pros and cons of surgically removing the prostate. In fairness to doctors whose livelihood is performing prostate surgery, they aren't wantonly practicing bad medicine. They undoubtedly believe they are saving lives. They might minimize the effectiveness of other procedures only because they aren't familiar with them. While others may see them as biased in favor of their own treatment, they see themselves conducting their profession to the best of their ability. Besides, not treating disease — active surveillance — just may not sit right. After all, doctors are trained to treat disease, not watch it! Then there's the reality of today's legal system: If a surgeon doesn't recommend surgery, a patient could sue the doctor if the cancer spreads or if another treatment goes wrong.

Which brings me back to the original offer: Let's make a deal! Only now, the deal is different. All I'm asking is that you read this book.

This book sets the record straight for you. You'll hear all the incredible facts about the medical politics that have resulted in hundreds of thousands of men getting needless surgery that has left a majority of them with partial or permanent disabilities involving incontinence and impotence. You'll learn about everything that can go wrong with the prostate, and you'll have the information you need to learn about treatment options — the facts you should be getting from your doctor. You'll also get practical and useful advice on lifestyle changes that can help prevent or perhaps delay prostate problems. And you'll learn things that may help slow the progression of disease you may already have. Then, you'll be armed with the facts you need to intelligently discuss treatment options with your doctor and make informed decisions.

No catches.

Nothing to do in return.

It's a deal I trust you'll be glad to make.

Frank K. Wood, Publisher

Debora Yost, Editor

P.S. Here's the rest of Rick's story:

As for my friend Rick, he got a second opinion from another oncologist and found out his prostate cancer was borderline between early-stage and intermediate-stage. He also found out that nerve-sparing surgery was impossible because of the location of the cancer — something, he was told, the diagnosing urologist had to have known. "He lied to you," the second opinion doctor candidly said. Rick opted to have brachytherapy. Twenty-four hours later, he and his wife were out for dinner as if nothing as dour as cancer treatment had taken place. That was nearly 10 years ago, and today Rick is in great health with no signs of recurring prostate disease. He never saw the doctor who diagnosed his disease again.

Part 1

You and your prostate

The prostate and the PSA: what men must know NOW

First, do no harm.
    --Hippocrates, the Father of Medicine

The PSA test is "a hugely expensive public health disaster," stated Richard J. Ablin, Ph.D., in a *New York Times* editorial in March 2010. That's a mighty powerful statement when you consider Dr. Ablin is the man who discovered PSA.

PSA is the acronym for prostate-specific antigen, an enzyme in the prostate gland that escapes into the bloodstream when there's something amiss in the gland that routinely lubricates the passage of sperm. It was an important discovery back in 1970 because the antigen tips off doctors that tumors are recurring in men who have been treated for prostate cancer. But in 1994, the U.S. Food and Drug Administration (FDA), based on scant evidence, approved the PSA test to screen for previously undetected prostate cancer. Doctors hastily embraced it as a simple, no-harm-done addition to the routine blood tests conducted during a man's annual physical examination. As it has turned out, the harm has been enormous.

Over the next decade and a half, shocking things happened in the annals of prostate health. The incidence of early-stage prostate cancer made a dramatic rise, deaths from late-stage prostate disease took a dive, and nearly a million healthy men with elevated PSAs but no symptoms of disease were scared into unnecessary radical surgery to have their prostates removed. This usually unnecessary surgery has left the majority of them struggling with a lifetime of impotence and incontinence. As a result, the PSA test has become one of the hottest and most contentious medical controversies of modern times.

Early detection. Fewer deaths. Shouldn't this be a good thing? Not when you consider that the majority of men with low-risk, early-stage cancer to this day are having risky surgery with life-altering consequences for a disease that probably would have never been a threat to them throughout their lifetime. In other words, a man who is lucky enough to reach old age is more likely to die with prostate cancer than from prostate cancer.

The U.S. Preventive Services Task Force (USPSTF) is an independent group of medical experts — family physicians, nurses, and specialists — who review a broad range of preventive health care tests and treatments. They then make recommendations based on their evaluations.

This well-respected panel already recommends against routine PSA tests for older men. They say if you're over 75 or if your life expectancy is less than 10 years, there is little to no benefit in detecting and treating prostate cancer. The harms, they say, outweigh the benefits.

Now they've released a new recommendation on PSA testing based on several trials done in Europe and in the United States. Two of these trials, reported in *The New England Journal of Medicine*, identified overwhelming evidence that, due to widespread PSA testing, prostate cancer is grossly overdiagnosed and overtreated.

In an interview for the *New York Times*, Dr. Peter B. Bach, of Memorial Sloan-Kettering Cancer Center, interpreted the findings of one of these studies. According to Bach, if he had a PSA test that led to a positive biopsy for prostate cancer, and then underwent treatment, there is a 49 in 50 chance the cancer was never life-threatening in the first place.

The USPSTF concludes that PSA screening in healthy men does not save lives and can result, instead, in unnecessary treatments that leave men with infections, impotence, and/or incontinence. This recommendation, however, does not apply to men suspected of having prostate cancer.

Too much, too fast

The problem with PSA screening is that it can detect slow-growing cancer cells that would never be a lifetime threat to even a young man. Well-documented evidence shows that 56 percent of cancers detected through a PSA test are low-risk, early-stage cancer, meaning they're unlikely to ever pose a threat to life or longevity. Yet 90 percent of men who get this diagnosis are electing to have major surgery with potentially life-altering consequences instead of a proven-to-be-safe alternative. Having no treatment, known as active surveillance, is a viable option that calls for vigilant checkups and postpones treatment to a time when the disease starts advancing. For many men, that time will never come.

Why are so many men willing to jump into surgery that has no greater potential to extend their life than doing nothing? Because it's the treatment most recommended by doctors. Despite the widely known fact that prostate cancer treatments cause "significant harms, including erectile dysfunction and urinary incontinence in many patients, many physicians continue to believe that the benefits of immediately treating PSA-detected prostate cancer outweigh the risks of delayed or no treatment," reported the Agency for Health-care Research and Quality in *Annals of Internal Medicine*. In the minds of the growing number of critics of PSA testing, this type of overtreatment is tantamount to mistreatment.

An FDA mistake

The U.S. Food and Drug Administration (FDA) approved the PSA test as a screening test for prostate cancer based on a study that showed it could detect 3.8 percent of cancers, which was a better rate than the current method used at the time, a digital rectal exam.

"The FDA should never have approved the PSA test as a screening test to detect prostate cancer," says Richard J. Ablin, the man who discovered PSA but did not develop the test. "It was a big mistake."

The remarkable outcome of active surveillance

To prove the point that active surveillance is a safe, sensible, and viable option for many men, Laurence J. Klotz, M.D., a Canadian researcher who is considered a visionary in his field, recruited 300 men with either low-risk or intermediate-risk prostate cancer who agreed to forgo treatment in favor of actively monitoring their disease. Their only treatment over the next five and a half years was a quarterly PSA test and a digital rectal exam. The physical exam, the only prostate cancer screener that was available prior to the PSA blood test, can detect a suspicious nodule by feel.

During the five and a half years, only 15 percent of the men ended up getting treated because their disease had advanced, and another 12 percent decided they wanted to get treated even though their disease had not changed. Two men with rapidly rising PSAs died from prostate cancer, despite immediate treatment. However, none of the other men, including those who eventually needed treatment, developed life-threatening metastatic disease during this time. Most of the men in this study were able to avoid the life-changing side effects of prostate surgery.

As a result of this study, the first Conference of Active Surveillance was called and attended by more than 200 of the world's leading experts in prostate cancer. The doctors agreed that if the basic requirements of low-risk disease were met, men of all ages could safely undergo active surveillance and delay treatment until increased risk showed a need for action, possibly avoiding treatment altogether. The conference resulted in a specific list of guidelines that doctors around the world could follow to safely monitor their patients with early prostate cancer and avoid immediately jumping into possible life-altering treatment.

The problem is the guidelines are often ignored in the drive for profit. Despite the continuing accumulation of evidence that active surveillance is sensible and safe, it's only lip service to many practicing urologists, says Anthony Zeitman, M.D., a radiation therapist from Massachusetts General Hospital. "The concept of active surveillance with selective therapy is taking root, and yet there is a paradox," he said in an editorial in the *British Journal of Urology*. "What is respectfully acknowledged at major medical meetings is not, in the daily reality of the clinic, being applied to patients. Indeed, the proportion of men being managed conservatively is actually declining."

Despite evidence of overdiagnosis and overtreatment and a cry from the American Cancer Society for surgeons to back off from aggressive treatment, too many men are being wheeled into operating rooms for unnecessary surgery. It has caused the most-informed and biggest opponents of aggressive treatment to throw up their arms and call for putting an end to using the PSA as a screening test to detect prostate cancer. And that includes a regretful Dr. Ablin. "I never dreamed that my discovery four decades ago would lead to such a profit-driven public health disaster," he says. "The medical community must confront reality and stop the inappropriate use of PSA screening."

The PSA test, says Dr. Ablin, "is hardly more effective than a coin toss. As I've been trying to make clear for many years now, PSA testing can't detect prostate cancer and, more important, it can't distinguish between the two types of prostate cancer — the one that will kill you and the one that won't."

Misinformed patients, greedy doctors

It helps to understand what's gone wrong when you consider the unusual dichotomy of prostate cancer. Urologists dominate the field of prostate cancer. This is the only kind of cancer in which this is the case. When a mammogram shows a lump or a physician detects a suspicious nodule elsewhere on the body, the patient is sent to an oncologist, a cancer specialist, for diagnosis and treatment. Oncologists have knowledge of a broad range of treatments in their field of specialty. However, when PSA rises, the family physician refers his patient to a urologist. Urologists are surgeons. They spend a great amount of personal time and money learning the very difficult surgery of removing the prostate. It's what they know how to do and the way they make their livelihood. They believe in what they are doing and trust that it saves lives. Studies show that, particularly where prostate cancer is concerned, most doctors recommend the treatment they are trained to perform. And more often than not it is radical prostatectomy.

Surgeons cut, radiologists radiate. This is nothing new to medicine. Getting around a urologist, however, is tough because oncologists generally do not deal with early-stage prostate cancer and finding one who specializes in prostate cancer is rare. Of the 10,000 medical oncologists in the United States, less than 100 specialize in prostate cancer.

As the facts and statistics concerning overdiagnosis and overtreatment of prostate cancer started surfacing during the last few years, major health organizations such as the American Cancer Society and the American Urology Association, have been quietly urging doctors to stop pushing for immediate and aggressive treatment. However, there is no evidence that it is happening.

Proof is in the numbers

The incidence of prostate cancer has risen dramatically since the PSA test became a standard screening procedure more than 15 years ago. Death rates from the disease have also significantly declined by 31 percent.

This sounds like a good thing, but it's not from a statistical point of view. "A true increase in cancers should be accompanied by an increase in death rates," says Laurence Klotz, M.D. The falling death rate, he says, suggests that "overdiagnosis is accountable for a significant proportion of the additional cases."

Prior to PSA screening, a man had a one in 40 lifetime risk of getting prostate cancer and a 12 percent chance of dying from it. Today, one in six men will be diagnosed with prostate cancer and 3 percent will die from it.

A long-term European study involving 182,000 men found that for every one life saved, 47 have to undergo unnecessary radical surgery and 1,410 have to be tested. However, it's questionable if studies that show "lives saved" always accurately measure death rates from all causes that may be increased as a consequence of surgery.

Don't shoot the messenger

For all the turmoil the PSA test has created, it is really not the problem. "The problem is doctors and patients overreacting to the information

PSA supplies," says Mark Scholz, M.D., a prostatic oncologist, critic of aggressive treatment, and the author of the book *Invasion of the Prostate Snatchers.* "The solution is not less frequent PSA testing, but rather convincing physicians to use a more restrained approach to recommending biopsy in men with slight PSA increases, particularly when there may be other reasons besides cancer causing the PSA elevation."

There is no doubt that PSA testing could potentially be a good thing, if used sparingly and appropriately when risk of developing the disease or recurrence is elevated. As a screening for prostate cancer it has saved lives. In the years prior to the PSA test, the disease was rarely diagnosed before it started revealing symptoms that it had spread, usually to the bone. Today, thanks to the PSA test, a man rarely walks into a doctor's office with late-stage prostate cancer. Critics, however, will argue that 47 men have to sacrifice their prostate, and most likely their potency, to save one life — a life that might not be lost anyway, if active surveillance were used to spot those who will benefit the most from surgery or other treatment. They don't feel that these are good odds.

"That's 47 men who, in all likelihood, can no longer function sexually or stay out of the bathroom for long," says Dr. Ablin, a research professor of immunobiology at the University of Arizona College of Medicine.

As a test to monitor the recurrence of prostate disease in men who have already been treated — the reason for which the test was originally intended — it also is a proven lifesaver. An elevated PSA is a telltale sign that all the cancer was not caught during surgery or that undetected cancer escaped the prostate capsule. As long as men who've been treated continue to have their PSA monitored, more aggressive treatment can be implemented to help halt the disease as soon as a noticeable rise is detected.

The problem with PSA, Dr. Ablin points out, is that it is not a true biomarker for prostate cancer because it doesn't detect cancer. It can only detect that there is something going on in the prostate that just isn't right — and most often it is a sign that the prostate is enlarging, a condition called benign prostatic hyperplasia (BPH) that is a natural part of aging.

A rising PSA can also be a sign of an infection called prostatitis. Certain medications, including drugs for BPH and common over-the-counter ibuprofen, can elevate PSA. Blood levels of PSA also go on the rise for a few days after having sex.

Sometimes there simply is just no logical explanation for a high PSA. It's just as likely that a man with a low PSA reading can harbor dangerous cancer cells as it is for a perfectly healthy man with harmless cancerous cells to test with a high reading.

Nevertheless the test has come under critical scrutiny and some leading specialists are slowly turning away from recommending it to their patients. They feel less testing will lead to fewer biopsies and fewer biopsies means there will be less unnecessary treatment. Some specialists, including Dr. Ablin, argue that routine PSA testing should be stopped completely. They feel diagnosing early prostate cancer is of detrimental value to most men. They see no point in giving men the burden of knowing they have a cancer that is best left untouched.

Most experts doubt, however, that PSA screening will ever be stopped because special interest groups have too much to gain financially. Most likely the PSA test is here to stay until something better comes along to improve on it or replace it. Several possibilities have popped up in research laboratories but it could be years before they prove conclusive and get federal approval.

Early low-risk disease is harmless

So where does this leave you? It should leave you with the recognition that every man needs to be acutely aware that prostate health in the 21st century is mired in politics and it is in your own best interest to take charge of your care. Though the criticism of PSA testing is making a lot of noise in the medical community, the facts about its limitations and consequences are not filtering down to the people who matter most — the men with low-risk disease. Too many men are unaware that early, low-risk disease is harmless. "This is starting to change," says Dr. Ablin, "but it's moving way too slow."

That's where this book comes in. The following pages offer you need-to-know information, based on the latest scientific evidence, on prostate health — what can go wrong, how it goes wrong, and what you can do about it to guarantee the best possible outcome. It also offers advice, based on scientific findings, on the lifestyle practices, foods, and nutrients that will help keep your prostate healthy.

Why men don't choose active surveillance as the best option for early-stage cancer

Using information from one of the largest and most complete cancer databases in the U.S., a study published in the *Archives of Internal Medicine* concluded that 44 percent of men diagnosed with prostate cancer, but with PSA levels less than 4 and considered low-risk, still underwent radical prostatectomies.

It's a phenomenon that has a lot of experts baffled, including a group of researchers who wanted to get inside the minds of some of the men who made this decision. What they found out was no surprise: The men followed their doctor's advice that it was the right thing to do.

In the researchers' correspondence with 198 men from California, South Carolina, and Texas, the men revealed they decided to have surgery because they trusted their doctors. They said they believed radical prostatectomy was superior to all other treatments and they were not concerned about its side effects. (In reality, the five-year survival rate for low-risk cancer is the same as no treatment and all other treatments — 99 percent.) The researchers also discovered that 87 percent of doctors told these men that radical surgery was a viable option but only 6 percent discussed active surveillance as an option.

"The men misperceived the cure of prostatectomy to other options," the researchers said in the study, reported in *The American Journal of Managed Care*. "There appears to be biases influencing a man's decision."

"Many men," noted the researchers, "have limited access to or a poor understanding of the evidence regarding management options" for low-risk, early-stage prostate cancer. They recommended that policymakers and clinicians do a better job of improving a man's understanding of prostate cancer and the ramifications of treatment options.

PSA: knowing the *real* score

The PSA test is far from perfect as a screening test for prostate cancer. It can indicate cancer when there is none and miss life-threatening disease. However, these are not the reasons why many experts believe the test should be shelved for routine testing and dismissed as a medical mistake. After all, no medical test is perfect. Critics of using the PSA test, a simple blood test that detects levels of prostate-specific antigen, to screen for prostate cancer oppose it because of what it cannot do and what has happened as a result.

"First, the test is not cancer-specific, meaning it can detect something is happening in the prostate but it doesn't have to be cancer," says Richard J. Ablin, Ph.D., research professor of immunobiology and pathology at the University of Arizona College of Medicine and the researcher who discovered PSA in 1970. "Second, the PSA test cannot distinguish tumor cells that are normal, benign, or malignant. Third, prostate cancer is an age-related disease. If you did biopsies on a totally random group of older men between the ages of 60 and 70, you'd find that 65 percent or more of them have prostate cancer." In other words, having cancer cells in the prostate gland is normal for most men over 60. However, Dr.

> "If you did biopsies on a totally random group of older men between the ages of 60 and 70, you'd find that 65 percent or more of them have prostate cancer. It doesn't mean, though, that you should be taking out their prostates."

Ablin adds, "It doesn't mean, though, that you should be taking out their prostates."

But prostate removal is exactly what's been happening. Too many operations have been performed on men who, if they had never been tested, could have continued living a healthy, normal life oblivious to the fact that they have cancer roaming in their prostate, just like Dr. Ablin's hypothetical group of 60- to 70-year-olds.

It's like the difference between a smoke alarm and a fire alarm, he says. "The PSA test is like a smoke alarm, but doctors and patients react like it's a fire alarm."

Dr. Ablin likes to draw a comparison of prostate cancer to an open box containing turtles and rabbits. "The turtles will just keep roaming around the box (the prostate) forever going nowhere. These are the harmless cancer cells. The rabbits might stay put for a while then suddenly jump out of the box. These are the aggressive, malignant tumors that escape the prostate and are life-threatening."

This is the conundrum that is prostate cancer. Nobody has yet been able to distinguish which tumors are harmless and which are potentially deadly. "All we know is that there are a lot more turtles than rabbits," says Dr. Ablin. Until that happens, there are going to be a lot more false fire alarms.

Benefits, limitations, and uncertainties

PSA is a protein molecule that measures an enzyme produced almost exclusively by cells in the prostate gland. PSA is secreted during ejaculation into the prostatic ducts that empty into the urethra. It liquefies semen and promotes the release of sperm. Normally, there are only very small amounts of PSA in the blood, though the level can vary depending on the size of the prostate gland. An abnormality in the prostate can disrupt the normal architecture of the gland and create an opening for PSA to pass into the bloodstream. This is what is detected on a PSA screening test. When levels of PSA are high, it is a sign of something wrong.

The weakness of the test is that it can't tell what is wrong. When a screening test detects a high PSA or a rising PSA, the next step is a biopsy, which can be painful and carries its own set of risk factors. (You'll read all about a prostate biopsy and how it's done on page 96). It turns out that about 50 percent of the time, a high PSA is due to an enlarged prostate. A larger prostate will naturally and normally produce more antigen. Anywhere from 20 to 40 percent of the time, the reason for a high PSA is cancer. Ten to 30 percent of the time, the reason for a high PSA is an infection or the reason is unknown. The test also carries a high rate of false positives — meaning it detected something wrong but nothing can be found — and an even higher rate of false negatives — meaning it didn't find cancer when it should have. PSA can also fluctuate substantially from day to day for no apparent reason.

Researchers were hoping that the issue over the benefits versus the risks of having a PSA screening test would be resolved with the results of two major long-term studies. The studies were published around the same time in the spring of 2010 in *The New England Journal of Medicine*. One study, conducted in Europe and involving 182,000 men, concluded the screening reduced deaths from prostate cancer by 20 percent. Remember, such studies often have biases that minimize deaths from other causes possibly related to reduced vitality as a consequence of prostate surgery. The study also found that 1,410 men had to be screened and 47 men subjected to unnecessary surgery in order to save one life.

The other study, involving 76,693 American men, found that screening did not save lives. A third study, also conducted in Europe and published a few months later in *Lancet Oncology*, found the risk of death in men who got screened and didn't get screened was about equal.

The contradictory findings in *The New England Journal of Medicine* studies fueled controversy with both opponents and proponents of screening claiming the study that didn't reflect their point of view was flawed. These two studies, however, made worldwide headlines because they captured the interest of the press for a different reason. The studies proved that the PSA test, whether it saves lives or not, leads to overdiagnosis and overtreatment of prostate cancer. That fueled the fire even more.

There is no magic number

PSA is measured in nanograms per milliliter (ng/mL), so when you get your test results back it can read anywhere from 0.1 ng/mL to 10 ng/mL to 20 ng/mL or even higher.

The American Cancer Society (ACS) has established 4 ng/mL as the threshold that divides safe from suspicious, but concedes that there is "no true cutoff point that distinguishes cancer from noncancer." Some European countries consider 3 ng/mL to be a safer threshold. However, studies have found detectable cancer cells approximately 40 percent of the time at PSA levels of 3 and 4.

The ACS counsels doctors to consider a PSA range of 2.5 to 4 to be an "indeterminate range," particularly for men who have no other risk factors for the disease.

Where's the informed consent that's truly informed?

The controversy over the PSA test, which has spread worldwide, isn't going to stop soon. In response to the USPSTF recommendations, the American Cancer Society (ACS) acknowledged this is a complex issue and urge men to become heavily involved in the decision to get screened for prostate cancer.

"It has been estimated that between 23 and 42 percent of screen-detected cancers would have never been diagnosed in the absence of screening," noted the ACS in issuing their screening guidelines to doctors, meaning the cancers were not significant enough to warrant action. "This degree of overdiagnosis and the associated overtreatment of invasive disease appears to be greater than for any other cancer for which routine screening currently occurs."

The guidelines say doctors have "an ethical mandate" to make sure patients understand "the benefits, limitations, and uncertainties related to screening for prostate cancer" before a drop of blood is drawn. Screening, say the guidelines, should be an informed and shared decision between doctor and patient.

Screening is defined as performing a medical intervention on a healthy individual who shows no signs or symptoms of having the disease that the test is designed to detect. In light of the controversy surrounding the test and its ramifications when PSA tests high, the guidelines remind doctors of the medical doctrine of *primum non nocere* — "First, do no harm."

"When the evidence is not clear that the benefits of screening outweigh the risk, an individual's values and preferences must be factored into the screening decision," say the guidelines. "In light of the uncertain balance between benefits and risk of prostate cancer screening, it is vital to involve men in the decision whether to screen."

Informed and shared decision making means that before you agree to or decline to have the test, your doctor should:

- explain the basic nature of how prostate cancer develops and other aspects of the disease.

- explain the uncertainties, risks, limitations, and potential benefits associated with screening, or choosing not to be screened.

- consider your personal feelings and preferences concerning screening.

- help you make an informed decision without bias and personal considerations if you can't or do not want to decide on your own.

So how's it going? If a survey conducted by the National Survey of Medical Decisions is any indication, it's not going well at all. The survey, which was reported in *Annals of Internal Medicine* and involved 3,010 men, found that discussions between doctors and men were not balanced, with doctors emphasizing the benefits of testing and, in many cases, not disclosing the cons. No discussion took place at all 30 percent of the time before the doctor wrote the prescription for the test — "a disconcerting finding," noted the researchers. Doctors also did not engage men to discuss their personal preference about testing.

When conversations did take place, the researchers found that the benefits of testing were explained 70 percent of the time but the negative aspects of the screening were explained only 30 percent of the time. Most of the men in the survey reported that their doctor thought favorably of the test and recommended it. Nearly 80 percent of the men who discussed screening with their doctor proceeded with the test.

Curiously, 90 percent of the men who engaged in a PSA conversation with their doctors felt the test was well-explained and 58 percent said they felt "very knowledgeable" about testing. Apparently this turned out not to be the case. When the researchers asked these men three questions they should have been able to answer as a result of shared decision making, half didn't even answer one question correctly.

The researchers concluded that "these discussions — when held — did not meet the criteria for shared decision making. Our findings suggest that patients need a greater level of involvement in screening discussions and to be better informed about prostate cancer screening."

Need-to-know information

In a discussion of PSA screening, your doctor should let you know the following.

- Screening with a PSA blood test alone or in conjunction with a digital rectal examination can detect cancer at an earlier stage than if no screening is performed.

- If cancer is detected as a result of screening, it currently is not possible to predict who will benefit from treatment.

- Most cancer detected through screening does not require immediate treatment. There are proven treatment methods other than surgery.

- There are many men who qualify for no treatment, but it requires continued vigilant testing and medical visits to keep check on the status of the cancer.

- The risks of treatment are substantial and can include sexual, urinary, and bowel dysfunction, depending on the treatment. These problems can be minimal or significant, permanent or temporary, also depending on the treatment.

- Evidence is not conclusive if screening reduces the risk of dying from the cancer.

- The PSA test can produce false positives, meaning that men without cancer but with abnormal results will be needlessly subjected to other invasive tests. It can also produce false-negative results, meaning that significant cancer may be missed.

- Abnormal screening results call for a biopsy to determine if the abnormal reading indicates cancer. Biopsies can be painful and can lead to complications including bleeding and infection. A biopsy can also miss finding cancer.

- Evidence is conflicting and experts do not agree on the value of screening.

When less testing means more

Reducing the frequency of PSA screening can reduce the number of men who lose their prostate to unnecessary surgery.

Screening every two years instead of annually would reduce the number of tests and unnecessary surgery by 50 percent without any decrease in lives saved, according to three different statistical analyses.

In the large European study that found screening reduced the risk of death by 20 percent, many of the 182,000 men who participated in the study were screened only every four years.

To test ... or not

The decision whether and when to get a screening test for prostate cancer is, in theory, up to you. However, in many situations, you may not be asked if you want to have the PSA test. You must be proactive and tell your doctor to omit the test if you don't want to have it, since it is often part of a battery of other routine blood tests. It is a highly individualized decision to forgo the test.

The ACS cites a few examples in which the decision to have the test is more or less clear-cut: If you're the kind of man who places a high value on finding cancer early and you're willing to undergo perhaps unnecessary surgery despite the risk of life-altering side effects, then screening is for you. On the other hand, if you place a higher value on protecting your sexuality and avoiding other issues that may affect your quality of life, then you might want to avoid screening.

For most men, however, the decision isn't so black or white. There are other important factors that should be considered.

Go with a doctor you can trust. "The screening decision is made best in partnership with a trusted source of regular care," advises the ACS. It's critical to your future well-being that you understand the pros and cons of screening. A PSA screening test is covered by virtually all insurance companies, so it is in your best interest to see a personal physician who can offer you the appropriate counseling rather than going to a large-scale community-based screening program that promotes screening.

If you see a private doctor who doesn't offer you information on the pros and cons of screening, then ask questions starting with, What are the pros and cons of getting this screening test? If the doctor doesn't take the time to discuss them with you and answer your other questions, see another doctor. It is important that you make an informed decision rather than automatically submit to a test that could open the door to a series of events that would have turned you off from the start.

Consider your age. Prostate cancer is an age-related disease and risk rises with each decade of life. Nevertheless, because prostate cancer is a slow-growing disease, most experts agree that a diagnosis of prostate cancer is of no value to men after the age of 75. This is based on statistics that show that 50 percent of men at age 75 do not have longevity beyond 10 more years. That said, every man is different. There are men in their 70s in excellent health who feel and look like they're in the prime of their life. If this is you, then the decision to screen or continue screening should be decided in consultation with your doctor.

The ACS does not consider screening necessary for healthy men at average risk for prostate cancer until the age of 50.

Know your family history. There's speculation that prostate cancer runs in families. The ACS recommends screening at age 45 for men with a first-degree relative, meaning a father or brother, who had prostate cancer. For men who have multiple first-degree relatives diagnosed with prostate cancer before the age of 65, the ACS recommends they begin discussions with their doctor about screening at the age of 40.

Take your race into consideration. The rate of prostate cancer in the United States is one of the highest in the world, largely due to the fact that black men have a 50 percent higher incidence of prostate cancer than white men. For this reason, the ACS recommends black men consider screening starting at age 45.

Factor in your state of health. You're a perfectly happy, healthy, in-shape, middle-aged guy who doesn't give much thought to the routine blood work that is done at the yearly physical. Then, before you can fully process what's happening, you're being wheeled into an operating room to have your prostate removed because your PSA reading was over 4. This is a scenario that has been played out among too many men — and one you should avoid. When you have the PSA discussion with your doctor, also have a discussion on what should happen if the test shows you have low-risk cancer.

By the same token, if you are in poor health or if you have a chronic disease that has a likelihood of shortening your lifespan, is there any value of adding slow-growing prostate cancer to your list of woes? For example, the ACS does not recommend screening will benefit men with moderate-to-severe chronic obstructive pulmonary disease, end-stage renal disease, moderate-to-severe dementia, life-limiting cancer, or severe congestive heart failure.

Don't count out testing permanently. If you decide against screening, don't rule it out forever simply based on the shortcomings of the PSA test. There is a lot of research currently taking place on alternative tests and on ways to make the current PSA test more reliable. During your yearly checkups ask your doctor what progress has been made that reduces the uncertainties regarding early detection of prostate cancer.

How well-informed are you?

If your doctor has a thorough discussion with you about the pros and cons of having a PSA screening test, you should know the correct answers to these three questions:

1. Of every 100 men, about how many do you think will die of prostate cancer?

2. Of 100 men, about how many will be diagnosed as having prostate cancer at some time in their lives?

3. For every 100 times a PSA test result suggests the need for further testing, about how many times does it turn out to be cancer?

According to results from the National Survey of Medical Decisions, when researchers posed these questions to men who thought that their doctors had advised them completely about the pros and cons of PSA screening, nearly half didn't answer any of the questions correctly. What about you?

For the answers, see page 341.

What to do after your PSA test

Every man is different. There are men who are getting screened because they should and there are men who want to get screened because they worry about cancer. There are even men who still think there is no harm in having a simple blood test, so they agree to it without thought. Whatever your reason for deciding on a PSA screening test, know what you're going to do with the information when the results come back. It is essential that you understand what the numbers mean, says Dr. Ablin. You should also know how to interpret your results and how you'll act on them.

Get a baseline — then do nothing. The baseline of any screening test is the number by which all other results are measured. Your baseline is the result of your first test. "Write the number down, write your age down, and keep it," says Dr. Ablin. "Never overreact to the first number. I know cases of too many men who underwent surgery because their first reading was high. This is wrong. Unless the number is in the high double digits, there is no reason to react like this."

Ask for a retest. If your first test results are high or the number seems out of character for your age and state of health, ask for a retest before reacting. "The number of false positives is very high," says Dr. Ablin. You should also get a retest before agreeing to undergo a biopsy.

Check for the size. At least 50 percent of the time, a rising PSA is due to an enlarged prostate. You don't have to go through a painful and risky biopsy to find this out. An easy-to-perform ultrasound can detect the size of the prostate. Ask your doctor about having this test before consenting to a biopsy.

Be like a turtle. Prostate cancer is the tortoise of cancers. In all but very rare cases it's not going to go anywhere fast. The key to understanding PSA is its doubling time. Only when it doubles too fast does it indicate trouble.

"If it goes from a 2 to a 4 in a few years or even a year, it's not a concern. If it goes from a 2 to a 4 in three months, it is a concern," says Dr. Ablin. "If your PSA is rising, ask to have it checked again in a few months before overreacting."

Remember, there is nothing significant about the number 4. Even though the ACS has selected 4 as the threshold for doctors to consider medical intervention, the number is totally arbitrary. "Cancer cells are found in men with a PSA under 4," says Dr. Ablin. "It just means these cells are nonthreatening. Don't panic if your PSA hits 4. Ask for a retest a few months down the line."

Check in with your emotions. Approximately 1.5 million American men between the ages of 40 and 69 are walking around with a PSA greater than 4. Doing so can be stressful and some men are better at handling it than others. For some men, getting a PSA test and just waiting for results raises anxiety.

One study of men whose PSA tests turned out to be a false positive, meaning the diagnosis of cancer turned out to be an error, had increased anxiety that lasted for a full year after the mistake was discovered. Anxiety was measured by the amount of the stress hormone cortisol in the blood. Another study found anxiety among men with a high PSA who were waiting for the results of their biopsy was 49 percent greater than normal.

Anxiety is the major side effect of screening, a burden you should also consider prior to testing. Other side effects are the same as with any other blood test and include a small risk of bruising, dizziness, and fainting.

Don't miss a test if you've been treated for cancer. The PSA test was originally designed for — and works best in — men who've been treated for prostate cancer. "When your prostate is taken out you shouldn't have any PSA reading," says Dr. Ablin. If a reading is detected, it's a sign that the cancer is recurring. Doctors will look at its doubling time to see how aggressive the cancer is. In this case, it is imperative that men keep up with their testing.

Age 75 with a PSA of 3 — you're safe!

Studies involving thousands of men found there was zero risk of ever having life-threatening prostate cancer if they matched this criteria: They were at least age 75 with a PSA of 3 or less.

The two sides to this story

Proponents of PSA as a screening test point to its justifiable benefits:

- It is the single best predictor of the presence of prostate cancer that is currently available.

- It can detect prostate cancer five to 10 years earlier than a digital rectal exam in which a doctor can physically feel a tumor.

- The majority of cancers detected by PSA tests are curable.

- Getting a first prostate test, known as a baseline, at age 50 can help predict the risk of getting the cancer in the next 25 years.

Opponents of the test point to its obvious negative consequences:

- Screening can detect cancer cells that will never become harmful to a man in his lifetime.

- Screening has resulted in overdiagnosis of the disease, which has resulted in hundreds of thousands of men having their prostate needlessly removed, leaving many of them with impotence, incontinence, and other quality-of-life issues.

- PSA screening was originally designed to test for recurring cancer in men who have been treated for prostate cancer, not as a test to find undetected cancer.

- It is not a true screening test because it does not detect cancer. Half of the time a rising PSA is caused by normal age-related prostate enlargement.

- The test has a high rate of false-positive and false-negative readings.

The party line

The American Cancer Society (ACS) prostate cancer screening guidelines, revised in 2011, say:

"The ACS recommends that asymptomatic men who have at least a 10-year life expectancy should have an opportunity to make an informed decision with their health care provider about whether to be screened for prostate cancer after receiving information about the uncertainties, risks, and potential benefits associated with prostate cancer screening. Prostate cancer screening should not occur without an informed decision-making process. Men at average risk should receive this information beginning at age 50 years. Men at higher risk, including African American men and men who have a first-degree relative (father or brother) diagnosed with prostate cancer before age 65 years, should receive this information beginning at age 45 years. Men at appreciably higher risk (multiple family members diagnosed with prostate cancer before age 65 years) should receive this information beginning at age 40 years. Men should either receive this information directly from their health care providers or be referred to reliable and culturally appropriate sources.

"Because prostate cancer grows slowly, those men without symptoms of prostate cancer who do not have a 10-year life expectancy should not be offered testing since they are not likely to benefit. Overall health status, and not age alone, is important when making decisions about screening.

"For men who are unable to decide, the screening decision can be left to the discretion of the health care provider, who should factor into the decision his or her knowledge of the patient's general health preferences and values."

The ACS also recommends:

- screening be conducted yearly if PSA is 2.5 or greater.

- screening be conducted every two years for a PSA under 2.5.

- screening can be performed in addition to or in the absence of a digital rectal exam.

- men at normal risk with a PSA of 4 or greater be referred for further evaluation or biopsy.

For men with a PSA between 2.5 and 4, doctors should consider risk factors including age, race, and family history, and perform a digital rectal exam before recommending a biopsy.

Part 2

When things go wrong

What can go wrong: common prostate problems

In life, the saying goes, two things are certain — taxes and death. In a man's life you could add another — prostate trouble.

Ninety percent of men will experience some type of prostate trouble in their lifetime, largely due to the unusual anatomy and habitat of the prostate gland. Picture a walnut. That's about the size and shape of your prostate. It sits snugly in your pelvis at the bottom of the bladder in front of the rectum and behind the base of the penis — a most unfortunate location because, when trouble starts brewing here, it affects the whole neighborhood.

The prostate gland is ground zero of the male reproductive system, as it serves as the manufacturing plant and transportation terminal for semen. The prostate gland is also a protectorate of the urinary tract because the urethra — the delivery tube that serves as the one-way freeway for semen and urine — passes right through it. You might say that this is an unfortunate landscape for your plumbing, because any interruption in the flow of traffic can create biological chaos akin to a traffic jam on a California freeway.

The anatomy of the prostate

Physicians look at the prostate from the perspective of zones. The peripheral zone is the outermost zone and makes up 70 percent of the prostate. This is the area where cancer is most likely to develop and is the target for taking sample tissue during a biopsy. Because this area sits so close to the rectum, it is possible for doctors to detect a suspicious mass during a digital rectal exam.

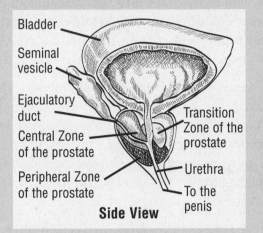

Side View

The central zone surrounds the ejaculatory duct and makes up about 25 percent of the prostate. Semen passes through this zone along the ejaculatory duct, where it meets up, in the form of a wishbone, with the urethra, which picks up the responsibility of delivering semen to its destination. Both benign prostatic hyperplasia (BPH) and cancer can develop in this area.

The smallest area is called the transition zone and makes up 5 percent of the gland. The urethra passes through this zone on its way from the bladder to the penis. BPH begins in the tissues within this zone. You can see how this would constrict the urethra and cause the urinary problems associated with BPH.

When a surgeon removes the prostate in a radical prostatectomy, the urethra must be reconnected to the bladder. Because the bladder is somewhat "soft," a small piece of the prostate is left intact to serve as a structure to keep the urethra securely in place. Most patients undergoing this surgery are not aware that, as a result of this, the prostate is not completely gone.

Unraveling the prostate puzzle

The prostate, which in large part is made up of muscle and fibrous tissue, is not really one large gland, but rather numerous little glands called acini that attach like clusters of grapes to the urethra. It works several jobs on your behalf. It manufactures prostatic fluid, a component of semen. It works like a traffic cop to keep urine and semen moving in the right direction and throws down the barricade so they'll never collide. Last, and certainly not least, it helps set off the sparks that pump semen from the seminal vesicles into the penis so you can experience the fireworks.

When you were born, the prostate was about the size of a pea and it stayed that way until you reached puberty. As you grew into manhood, your prostate went through a growth spurt of its own, reaching adult size around age 20. Then somewhere around age 25 or so, it started to grow again, ever so slowly. Considering a normal healthy prostate weighs about an ounce, we do mean slowly.

If you're lucky — and most men are not — this growth might not cause you any problems, or symptoms could be ever so slight that you'll never really take notice. More likely, though, by the time you reach your early 50s, that growth will start to impede urine flow through the urethra like freeway traffic forced into one lane in a construction zone. The first hint that it is also impinging on your life is when you start to notice that a visit to the bathroom isn't as easy as it used to be.

An enlarged prostate is not the only thing that can disrupt life in the gland of joy. The prostate's territorial rights to both the urinary tract and the erogenous zone leave this tiny gland vulnerable to a variety of infections. Then, of course, there's the much more serious threat no one wants to think about — prostate cancer. It's no wonder that there are some 50,000 urologists in the United States at the service of the prostate gland. Don't be too surprised if suddenly one day you find yourself taking your gland to meet one of them.

If and when it happens, here's a fact to help you keep your cool and your thought processes clear: Prostate disease is treatable and should cause only minimal inconvenience in your life, if you respond at the first sign of trouble. So check out the box *Symptoms of a sick prostate.* If you are experiencing any of them, make an appointment to see your doctor as soon as possible. The rest of this section tells you what can go wrong with the prostate, how a problem is diagnosed, the pros and cons of the many treatment options that are now available, and how to work with your doctor so your prostate can keep on working as nature intended.

Symptoms of a sick prostate

One or more of these symptoms could be a sign of prostate trouble:

- frequent or urgent urination
- slow or interrupted urine stream
- blood in the semen or urine
- difficulty starting to urinate
- difficulty emptying the bladder
- waking up at night to urinate*
- involuntary dribbling or urine spotting
- a great urge to urinate that results in only going a little bit
- painful urination
- bladder pain that is relieved by urinating
- painful intercourse or ejaculation
- pain in the perineum, the area between the penis and anus

Some of these symptoms can also be accompanied by:

- chills
- fever
- lower back pain

* Waking up at night with a full bladder may also be a consequence of lower testosterone levels with normal aging.

Benign prostatic hyperplasia:
your growing prostate

Benign prostatic hyperplasia, or BPH, is the technical name for one of the most common problems in men — an enlarged prostate. This abnormal growth occurs when normal healthy cells overpopulate and start to pile up in the tiniest place in the prostate known as the transition zone. Because the gland is muscular, it can resist the nudge from these cells, forcing them to push and bulge inward by pressing against the urethra. When you look at the illustration on page 35, you can see how this happens.

This stranglehold on the urethra is what BPH is all about. It causes any number of symptoms that can make urination difficult or downright painful.

BPH happens because the normal life-and-death cycle of healthy prostate cells goes grossly off-course. In a normal prostate, individual healthy cells die about every four months and are replaced by new healthy cells. In BPH, however, as healthy cells come to life, old cells hang in there. Before you know it, the prostate is operating with an overcapacity crowd. Just like in an overcrowded prison, these old cellmates can get a bit unruly. They gang up and form clusters called nodules that push their size around, making it harder and harder for the urethra to resist. When quarters get too tight, the urethra starts inching inward. That's when you start to take notice. The first sign may be a bladder that doesn't empty completely or a stream that tends to dribble. Or, you might feel a strong urge to urinate that cannot wait. It really starts messing with your life when you have to get up at night — often several times — to go to the bathroom, preventing a good night's sleep that you feel as fatigue and lethargy the next day. This can have such an impact on your health that doctors have a name for it — nocturia.

Why prostate cells run amok is not fully understood, but research suggests a combination of aging and androgens, the collective term for male hormones, are involved. As a man ages, his hormonal balance makes a shift. Active levels of testosterone in the blood decline, leaving a higher proportion of the female hormone estrogen, which is present in men in small amounts. Animal studies suggest that estrogen activates substances that make the prostate grow.

Another theory involves dihydrotestosterone (DHT), the active form of testosterone. Even though testosterone levels decline with age, older men continue to produce and accumulate large levels of DHT in the prostate. DHT is nine times more powerful than testosterone. Scientists have noted that men with enlarged prostates have high levels of DHT and men who do not produce DHT do not get BPH.

Genetics also appear to play a role, as the condition tends to run in families and is more common among black men than white men.

One in every four American men experiences BPH-related symptoms by the time they reach their mid-50s. By age 75, half of all American men experience some type of urinary discomfort related to BPH. By age 80, an estimated 20 to 30 percent of men experience symptoms severe enough to require minimally invasive treatment or surgery.

Lots of LUTS

BPH is not life-threatening, nor does it increase your risk of prostate cancer. Progression of the disease, however, is a guessing game. Some men are fortunate enough to never feel any discomfort or pain from BPH. For most men this is not the case. BPH typically evolves into some degree of lower urinary tract symptoms — what doctors refer to as LUTS. You can experience one, several, or even all of them. They are:

- a sudden and strong urge to urinate, called urinary urgency

- the sensation that the bladder isn't completely empty

- nocturia — sleep disturbances caused by the need to urinate

- a weak or erratic stream

- intermittent — stopping and starting — urine flow

- an occasional, or more frequent, little leak or two

- a sensation of fullness behind the scrotum and in front of the rectum

Lots of LUTS can affect quality of life. Their severity and your tolerance to them help determine your course of treatment. Even if you are able to grin and bear them all, you should not ignore the symptoms of BPH. The pressure it puts on the urethra can lead to more pressing problems down the line.

Nocturia: risky business

Having a prostate that gets you up in the middle of the night to go to the bathroom is more than a nuisance. It's also a real threat to life and limb.

Nocturia is a condition defined as having to get up two or more times during the night to urinate. The incidence rises with age and fading health.

It is one of the most disturbing symptoms of BPH. While BPH in itself is not life-threatening, nocturia can be.

Two studies, one in Massachusetts and the other in Japan, found an increased risk of premature death among people with nocturia compared to people who slept through the night. Although no single cause of death was cited in the studies, researchers took a wild guess — accidental falls while going from bedroom to bathroom.

Nocturia is also frequently caused by lower testosterone levels associated with aging. Relatively high testosterone levels early in life tend to reduce the production of urine while asleep. Having to get up with a full bladder in the middle of the night without other symptoms of BPH may simply be a consequence of having low testosterone levels.

One thing leads to another

BPH doesn't just affect the prostate. It can create changes in the bladder. When the prostate constricts the urethra, the smooth muscle wall of the bladder must contract more to expel urine. These stronger contractions cause the bladder wall to thicken, which means there is less room to accumulate and hold urine. Over time, the bladder is capable of holding less and less urine, meaning you're taking more frequent trips to the bathroom. As the cellular noose around the urethra gets tighter, the contractions that control urine don't always go with the flow, so to speak, and the bladder doesn't always empty completely, a condition called urinary retention.

Urinary retention can create its own set of problems. Urine left behind can cause the bladder to become overly sensitive to the point that you are unable to heed nature's call quickly enough — and before you know it, you're incontinent.

Sometimes you may not be able to urinate at all, a medical emergency called acute urinary retention. It is impossible to predict and usually occurs unexpectedly. Acute urinary retention is serious and considered a medical emergency requiring catheterization, a procedure in which a tube is inserted through the penis and into the bladder to force urine flow.

Urine that sits in the bladder is dangerous. It can become infected or lead to bladder stones. In rare instances, an overstressed bladder or bladder infection can lead to kidney damage.

The causes of acute urinary retention

It happens suddenly, unexpectedly, and for no known reason. There are a few things known to help contribute to an attack:

- alcohol
- antidepressants
- decongestants
- tranquilizers
- urinary tract infections

Diagnosing BPH

Oftentimes, the first clue that you have an enlarged prostate occurs when your doctor detects it through a digital rectal exam during your annual physical. When this happens, he or she will ask you a few questions concerning recent changes in urinary habits. If your doctor suspects that your urinary symptoms need medical attention, you'll most likely be referred to a urologist for further evaluation, diagnosis, and treatment.

The American Urology Association has come up with a handy seven-point questionnaire called the International Prostate Symptom Score (IPSS) that doctors use to help determine if you have BPH and assess its severity. It's also used to help guide treatment. You can take this quiz on your own and we'll show you how in just a moment. First, an important message.

Changes and troubles in your urinary department in and of themselves are not a diagnosis of BPH, even if your doctor feels an enlargement. There are medical conditions that can mimic BPH. They include:

- bladder stones, the buildup of hard minerals

- prostatitis, an infection of the prostate gland

- urethral stricture, an abnormal narrowing of the urethra caused by an injury or disease

- neurogenic bladder, urinary dysfunction associated with the central nervous system as a result of injury or disease

- bladder outlet obstruction (BOO), a blockage at the base of the bladder that reduces or prevents the flow of urine to the urethra

- bladder or prostate cancer

Also, bladder habits change — that is, they can become more troublesome — with age, meaning you may unfortunately be saddled with urinary difficulties similar to BPH, but you're disease-free.

Help make your diagnosis

This seven-point questionnaire, called the International Prostate Symptom Score (IPSS), is used by doctors around the world to help determine the severity of BPH symptoms and determine the course of treatment. It's simple to take and easy to score.

Check the number that best describes your urinary habits during the past month.

During the last month, how often have you ...					
Not at all	Less than 1-in-5	Less than half the time	About half the time	More than half the time	Almost always
1. had the sensation of not emptying your bladder completely after you finished urinating?					
0 ○	1 ○	2 ○	3 ○	4 ○	5 ○
2. had to urinate again within two hours after you finished urinating?					
0 ○	1 ○	2 ○	3 ○	4 ○	5 ○
3. found you stopped and started several times when urinating?					
0 ○	1 ○	2 ○	3 ○	4 ○	5 ○
4. found it difficult to postpone urination?					
0 ○	1 ○	2 ○	3 ○	4 ○	5 ○
5. had a weak urinary stream?					
0 ○	1 ○	2 ○	3 ○	4 ○	5 ○
6. had to push or strain during urination?					
0 ○	1 ○	2 ○	3 ○	4 ○	5 ○

During the last month, how many times ...					
None	1 time	2 times	3 times	4 times	5 times or more
7. is your sleep interrupted at night because of the need to urinate?					
0 ○	1 ○	2 ○	3 ○	4 ○	5 ○

Now, add up the numbers you checked to get your total score.

Total score: _____

What your score means

The score measures the severity of these symptoms as follows:

1-7: Mild   8-19: Moderate   20-35: Severe

The American Urological Association recommends no treatment for mild symptoms, some type of treatment to alleviate moderate symptoms, and surgery to relieve severe symptoms.

What to expect from your urologist

When you see a urologist, he will do a medical history and a physical examination that includes a digital rectal exam, in which the doctor inserts a lubricated gloved finger into the rectum to feel if the prostate is enlarged. You'll be asked about any previous urinary problems, if you've ever had a catheter inserted, your sexual practices, and your use of medications. Certain decongestants and allergy medicines can mimic BPH or aggravate symptoms if you have BPH.

You will be asked the seven key IPSS questions. If your answers indicate that your symptoms are mild, a score of 1 to 7, the only test you'll probably need to confirm an enlarged prostate is a urinalysis, which is a microscopic examination of a urine sample. Your doctor may also order a PSA test. Men with BPH have higher than normal levels of circulating PSA. (PSA is controversial. You can read all about it and its limitations in Part 1.)

If your symptoms are moderate to severe, a score of 8 or higher, your doctor most likely will recommend one or more diagnostic tests to assess if BPH is adversely affecting your urinary tract, bladder, or kidneys in any way.

These are the tests that are commonly used to confirm and assess the severity of symptoms.

Cystometry. This test is used to evaluate problems with urination, urinary incontinence, urinary retention, and infection by assessing how efficiently the bladder fills and empties. During the test, the doctor will insert two small catheters through the urethra and into the bladder. One catheter fills the bladder with warm water, a saline solution, or carbon dioxide gas, while the other catheter records pressure changes in the bladder while it is being filled and emptied.

While the solution is going in, you'll be asked to describe the sensation of filling and any discomfort. When the bladder is full, you'll be asked to void.

Some men complain of some discomfort during the test. There is no special preparation needed and the only aftercare required is about an hour of relaxation. There is a slight risk of developing a urinary tract infection due to a tear of the urethral lining.

Uroflowmetry. This is a simple test used to detect if urine flow is normal or lagging. It involves urinating into an electronic device that measures the volume of urine excreted and the speed of the flow. No special preparation is required except you must have a full bladder when taking the test.

Ultrasound. This is a painless imaging test in which the technician presses a microphone-like device called a transducer against the skin of the lower abdomen. As the device passes over the skin it emits sound waves that reflect off the internal organs. It can detect structural abnormalities in the bladder and kidneys, such as stones, and estimates the size of the prostate. It can also determine the amount of residual urine in the bladder. This test is generally only performed on men with severe lower urinary tract symptoms.

Intravenous pyelography. Your doctor may order this test if he suspects your BPH is creating a blockage in your urinary tract or bladder. The test is an X-ray that involves injecting dye into a vein that circulates into these organs to search for a blockage. The only risk is a possible allergic reaction to the dye. You shouldn't have the test if you know you have an allergy to iodine.

Pressure-flow urodynamic study. This test is considered the gold standard for detecting a bladder outlet obstruction (BOO), which can occur in men with severe BPH. It involves placing a recording device in the bladder and sometimes the rectum to detect the difference in pressure between the bladder and rectum when bladder muscles contract. A high pressure accompanied by a low urine flow indicates BOO. Low pressure with a low urine flow is a sign of an abnormality in the bladder itself. The test can cause discomfort for a short time. In a few men, it may cause a urinary tract infection.

Your treatment options

Treatment for an enlarged prostate has come a long way since your grandfather's time when surgery was the only option. In your dad's day, drug therapy hit the market and is still one of the current commonly used treatments. In recent years, a variety of minimally invasive surgeries are proving to be more attractive options because they pose less risk, both to your overall health and your love life.

Science has made some major advances in treating BPH — there are many treatments from which to choose — but researchers have gotten nowhere in finding a cure for the disease. The only approach is to treat and mask the symptoms.

Having a range of choices, in a way, is a problem of its own. There is no one-size-fits-all treatment for BPH and they all have their share of risks, not the least of which are the possibilities of incontinence and sexual difficulties, including impotence and problems ejaculating. Also, every man experiences BPH in his own way and tolerates symptoms differently, so what's good for another man is not necessarily the best treatment for you.

Your doctor will generally advise you based on several factors.

- how bothersome your symptoms are, meaning how they are affecting your quality of life

- what studies indicate are the best options for your symptoms and general health

- the treatments your urologist has experience performing

- the anecdotal feedback from the men your doctor has previously treated, though this could be different from the way you'd feel and respond to the same treatment

If your IPSS indicates your symptoms are mild, you have the option of doing nothing until your symptoms get worse — and it's possible they never will. Men whose symptoms are at the top of the score card generally face the possibility of surgery, especially if drug therapy has not worked. It's the men in the middle — and that's the majority — who have the toughest decision. Should you wait and see how things go? Start taking drugs that you might have to take for the rest of your life? Try a minimally invasive procedure, which may or may not work over the long term?

There is no rule of thumb for what treatment is best for certain symptoms. In the end, it all comes down to individual preference, says Alan W. Partin, M.D., Ph.D., urologist-in-chief and director of the urology department at Johns Hopkins University School of Medicine. "Some men don't want to take drugs every day and want to have the minimally invasive therapy. Others want to take a pill along with their vitamins and avoid any procedure."

To decide the best treatment for you, discuss your symptoms with your doctor and be candid about your tolerance level. Ask about the risks and benefits of all procedures, even if he has little or no experience with them, and decide how you feel about them. Ask these important questions about each treatment.

- What are my chances of getting better?
- How much better will I get?
- What are the chances that the treatment will cause problems?
- How long will the treatment work?

Many doctors have access to video and computer programs that present the risks and benefits of different types of treatments in an easy-to-understand format. The programs feature men who've experienced good as well as bad outcomes after having prostate treatment. Some men find viewing computer or video programs gives them a clearer idea of which option they'd like to choose.

Colds, allergies, and prostate trouble

If you're taking over-the-counter medication for a cold or allergy, make sure you tell your doctor. Taking certain decongestants and antihistamines can mimic symptoms of an infected or enlarged prostate. They can also make symptoms worse in men who have these conditions.

Decongestants, such as pseudoephedrine (Sudafed) and diphenhydramine (Benadryl) belong to a class of drugs called adrenergics that exacerbate urinary symptoms by preventing muscles in the prostate and bladder neck from relaxing and allowing urine to flow freely.

When buying medicine for a cold or allergy, always check the label. Products that could potentially cause problems for men with prostate trouble should carry a warning, so read the fine print.

There are stories of more than a few unfortunate men whose silence about medications they were taking has resulted in unnecessary prostate surgery.

Taking an active role in choosing your treatment is important. According to a five-year study supported by the Agency for Health Care Policy and Research, the best way to lower your chances of getting overtreated is to play an active role in deciding your own treatment. Most importantly, give yourself time to decide how you feel about your options.

These are the treatment options currently available for BPH and what recent research has found concerning their strengths, weaknesses, and effectiveness.

Watchful waiting

Watchful waiting is another way of saying "do nothing" and it is the option of choice for men who have yet to experience symptoms or do not find their symptoms bothersome. It means seeing your doctor once or twice a year for a checkup, and calling your doctor for an appointment if you start to have troublesome urinary problems.

Totally doing nothing at all, however, is not a good idea. The way you choose to live your life has an impact on your prostate health. While you are watchfully waiting you should make a conscious effort to do the following.

Adopt a healthy lifestyle. Out of all the conditions that affect your prostate, BPH is the one that responds best to changes, both big and small, that you make in your life. The type of lifestyle that complements a healthy prostate is detailed in Chapter 9.

Eat a low-fat diet. Studies show that the risk of BPH is highest in men who eat a high-fat diet and lowest in men who eat the least fat. Chapter 10 outlines all the tasty choices that have been scientifically found to be prostate-friendly.

Cut down on your drinking. We're not just talking alcohol here. Also limit caffeinated coffee, tea, and soft drinks. Caffeine tends to tighten the bladder neck, which makes it more difficult to urinate. Also, sip rather than guzzle and don't drink a lot at one time. To reduce the need to get up at night to urinate, try not to drink anything after 7 p.m. and always empty your bladder before going to bed.

Skip the spicy cuisines. Spicy foods can aggravate an enlarged prostate. If you notice more problems after you've eaten Mexican, Indian, or other spicy foods, avoid them.

Go when you gotta go. Take the time to urinate when it is convenient, even if there is no urge. For example, take advantage of intermission when at the theater or a concert. If you're headed for a long meeting, hit the men's room on the way. When you're out and about and see a public restroom, pause and make a visit.

Keep warm. If you're looking for an excuse to head south in the winter, you've got one. Cold weather can make urinary tract symptoms worse. Cold increases activity in the sympathetic nervous system, which causes increased smooth muscle tone within the prostate and makes it harder to urinate. Urinary retention is more likely to occur in the winter than the summer.

Have sex — often. It's the silver lining in having BPH. Ejaculating frequently helps make urination easier because it helps empty the prostate of secretions that can hamper urination.

Practice Kegel exercises to strengthen your sphincter. The sphincter is a ring of muscle that opens and closes to allow urine to escape from the bladder. Keeping this muscle taut with exercises known as Kegels can help prevent involuntary leakage. Kegels were originally developed to help women through pregnancy, but they work just as effectively in helping men with BPH.

Because the muscle you are exercising is internal, it can be difficult to isolate. The easiest way to learn how to perform Kegels is while urinating. Here's how. As soon as urine starts to flow make a contraction to slow flow. Hold for 10 seconds. Then make another contraction to stop. Hold for another 10 seconds. Repeat until you're finished.

Do Kegels while you're urinating only as practice. Kegels are not intended to be performed while going to the bathroom, as doing so can eventually weaken the muscle.

Once you get the feel for it, you can exercise your sphincter when it's at rest. Kegels can be done anywhere — while you're driving, when you're sitting at your desk working, or when relaxing in the evening watching television. Perform the exercise by doing 10 to 15 contractions three to five times a day.

Learn to relax. Stress can make an already difficult urinary problem worse. Nerves in the bladder neck and prostate are sensitive to adrenaline, the hormone that is released when you're under stress. Also, just as it is difficult to get an erection when you're feeling stressed, it is just as hard to urinate.

Get off your prostate. You sit on your prostate and that's not good. Take breaks if you're sitting at a desk all day. Stand when you can, rather than sit, such as when you're at the bar waiting for a table. If sitting irritates your enlarged prostate, get a pillow designed with a hole in the middle like a doughnut. This type of pillow was originally designed for people with hemorrhoids and can be purchased at a medical supply store.

Pedal with care. Bicycling can be a mixed blessing. It's associated with lower rates of prostate cancer in one study, perhaps because the bicycle seat massages the prostate while biking. But an improperly adjusted bicycle saddle or seat — one that is set too high, for instance — can damage the perineal area and cause problems with sexual function. Also, bicycling may sometimes aggravate prostatitis or inflammation of the gland.

Sitz it out. Sitz, which is German for seat, is a hot bath for soaking the pelvic area. Just fill the tub a few inches — enough to submerge yourself no higher than the belly button — with water that's hot to the touch but comfortable enough to sit in. Soak for 15 minutes. When symptoms are particularly aggravating, try taking a sitz bath three times a day.

Go herbal. Don't be surprised if your doctor asks if you'd like to try to control your symptoms and your enlarging prostate with herbs. Even mainstream medicine recognizes the merits of certain herbs and minerals for BPH, including African plum, beta-sitosterol, rye pollen extract, saw palmetto, and stinging nettle. You can read about these supplements and the effect they might have on your prostate in Chapter 11.

BPH in the bedroom

The average male with mild BPH should not have a problem with sexual performance. However, trouble in the bedroom can mount with the severity of symptoms — and it can go either way: premature ejaculation or problems having or maintaining an erection.

One study, reported in the *British Journal of Urology*, followed the love lives of 11,834 men and found that multiple lower urinary tract problems created more trouble with erectile dysfunction, premature ejaculation, or difficulty ejaculating. The researchers found that problems mounted as these factors came into play:

- an increase in severity of symptoms
- aging
- high blood pressure
- diabetes
- depression
- fear of leaking
- leaking while having sex

Another study examined the effect of BPH medications on sexual desire. It found that men taking alfuzosin (Uroxatral), doxazosin (Cardura), or terazosin (Hytrin) reported fewer problems getting erections than men taking the androgen suppressants dutasteride (Avodart) and finasteride (Proscar). They also had better ejaculations than men taking the alpha blocker tamsulosin (Flomax).

Managing BPH with medicine

The prostate is largely made up of two types of tissue with distinctly different jobs. The primary job of glandular tissue is to produce fluid involved in the production of semen. Smooth muscle tissue regulates the involuntary passage of fluids into the urethra. These systems mesh like clockwork until glandular tissue starts to grow and encroach on the urethra, making it difficult for smooth muscle tissue to stay in time. When urinary stream is slow or cut off, it is a sign of a smooth muscle contracting.

There are two types of prescription medications, each aimed at stopping the errant action of one of these tissues. Androgen suppressants, the common name for 5-alpha-reductase inhibitors, target glandular tissue and work by slowing its growth. Alpha blockers, the common term for alpha-1-adrenergic blockers, target smooth muscle and work by relaxing contractions so urine can flow.

Studies have found that taking prescription medication can help improve symptoms of BPH anywhere from 30 to 60 percent. How much your symptoms improve, however, depends on which tissue is causing you the most trouble and that's not always easy to figure out. Neither drug is effective for everyone, especially if you suffer from multiple issues, and both carry the risk of side effects that can impact your quality of life. More recent research shows that taking a combination of both might be better than taking either one alone.

There is a general belief that drug therapy is a lifetime decision because symptoms will start to come back if the medications are stopped.

Androgen suppressants

These drugs prevent glandular tissue from growing by stopping the action of 5-alpha-reductase, the enzyme responsible for converting the male sex hormone testosterone into dihydrotestosterone (DHT), which is linked to fueling prostate growth. There are two androgen suppressants on the market:

- dutasteride (Avodart)
- finasteride (Proscar)

Studies show they can reduce prostate size — and therefore release pressure on the urethra — from 20 to 30 percent. One major study, reported in the *British Journal of Urology International*, compared the effectiveness of one against the other and found them to be about equal. After taking the medication for one year, men experienced a 27 percent reduction in prostate size and their prostate symptom scores improved by 6.6 points.

Advantages. Studies show that taking androgen suppressants helps reduce the risk of acute urinary retention. In one study, finasteride reduced the risk by 55 percent after four years. Taking androgen suppressants has also been found to decrease the risk of needing surgery in the future.

Disadvantages. It can take three to six months to start feeling the effects of androgen suppressants and a year to feel the full effect.

Sexual side effects. From a quality-of-life perspective, they are severe, though the risk is small. Impotence occurs in 7 to 8 percent of men taking the drug and low libido affects 5 to 6 percent. There is also a risk of breast enlargement but it is less than 1 percent.

The ideal candidate. Androgen suppressants work best in men with large prostates — 50 percent or larger than normal size — with moderate to severe symptoms.

Drug reduces cancer risk

Dutasteride appears to have a two-for-one advantage. It can reduce the symptoms of BPH and help guard against prostate cancer, according to a study published in *The New England Journal of Medicine.*

Researchers put 6,729 men who were considered to be at high risk for prostate cancer on dutasteride or a placebo. After four years, fewer men taking the dutasteride got cancer than men taking the placebo. The drug reduced cancer risk by 23 percent.

> ## Pregnancy warning
>
> If you're taking androgen suppressants, keep the pills out of the way of pregnant women. Studies show that pregnant women who are exposed to crushed or broken androgen suppressants risk exposing their male fetuses to birth defects.

Baldness and BPH: connecting the follicles

What do male-pattern baldness and benign prostatic hyperplasia (BPH) have in common? Apparently a hormonal defect that leaves certain men at high risk for both.

Male-pattern baldness, which accounts for almost all hair loss in men, results from a genetic malfunction that causes hair follicles to shrink and eventually stop producing hair in the presence of dihydrotestosterone (DHT), the active form of the male hormone testosterone. Both men with male-pattern baldness and those with BPH have high levels of circulating DHT. The link is so strong that finasteride, the drug marketed under the brand name Proscar that helps shrink the prostate gland, is also marketed as Propecia, the drug that helps stop hair loss in more than 85 percent of men who take it. The only difference is that Proscar is a whole lot stronger than Propecia.

Scientists in Spain, suspecting a link between the two conditions, recruited 60 men with identical health factors and lifestyle patterns for a research study. None of the men had any known symptoms of BPH. The only obvious physical difference among them was that half the men had early-onset male-pattern baldness and the other half had a full head of hair.

To test their theory, the scientists used ultrasound, a painless noninvasive procedure, to measure the size of the men's prostates. They found that the balding men had enlarged prostates, which were an average of 34 percent larger than the men with a full head of hair. Another test confirmed that the balding men also were not urinating at full volume. Their urine volume was an average of 32 percent less than the guys with hair.

The scientific conclusion: The balding men all had BPH, but just didn't know it — yet.

"This study suggests that patients with male-pattern baldness should talk with their doctors about any urinary symptoms they may be experiencing so they can take preventive measures," the researchers concluded.

The benefit: Taking finasteride in the dose designed to treat BPH would offer a two-for-the-price-of-one approach. It could be a helpful solution for baldness and BPH. Just remember that side effects reducing male sexuality are a real risk of such drugs.

Alpha blockers

Originally developed to treat high blood pressure, these drugs relax smooth muscle tissue by blocking the nerve impulses that signal muscles to contract, making it easier to urinate. Alpha blockers have a big advantage over androgen suppressants because they go to work faster. Relief in the form of increased urinary flow, reduced urgency in the need to urinate, and fewer interruptions at night to go can be felt in just a few days.

There are several different alpha blockers on the market.

- alfuzosin (Uroxatral)
- doxazosin (Cardura)
- prazosin (Minipress)
- silodosin (Rapaflo)
- tamsulosin (Flomax)
- terazosin (Hytrin)

All have been found to be effective at relieving symptoms of BPH, according to a review published in *The Journal of Urology*. Men who took alfuzosin showed a 19 to 50 percent improvement on prostate symptom scores. Men taking doxazosin showed a 14 to 39 percent improvement, men taking tamsulosin improved 24 to 50 percent, and those taking terazosin improved 38 to 64 percent.

Advantages. In addition to bringing quick relief from symptoms, the symptoms might not return if you stop taking the drug. In one study, symptoms did not return within one year in 70 percent of men who stopped taking the drug. For men with high blood pressure, the drug may serve a dual purpose.

Disadvantages. Alpha blockers have a potentially greater negative impact on your sex life than androgen suppressants. Also, they can make certain sex-enhancing drugs ineffective. The medications involved are oral phosphodiesterase type 5 (PDE5) inhibitors — sildenafil (Viagra), tadalafil (Cialis), and vardenafil (Levitra).

Sexual side effects. The risk of retrograde ejaculation is 4 to 18 percent, erectile dysfunction is 5 to 16 percent, and reduced libido is 3 to 6 percent. Of all the brands, silodosin is most likely to cause retrograde ejaculation.

The ideal candidate. Best for men with smaller prostates who have moderate to severe symptoms.

Combination drug therapy

Two drugs. Two different approaches to relieving debilitating BPH. Obviously, it's not much of a stretch to wonder if each drug is effective on its own, would taking two work even better?

It appears that it does, according to two major studies involving thousands of men.

The first study, called the Medical Therapy of Prostatic Symptoms (MTOPS), involved 3,047 men with BPH who received either the alpha blocker doxazosin, the androgen suppressant finasteride, a combination of the two, or a placebo. After 4½ years, the men taking the combination drug were 66 percent less likely to experience an increase in symptoms than men taking the placebo. By comparison, doxazosin alone reduced risk by 39 percent and finasteride by 34 percent.

The second study, called CombAT for the combination of dutasteride (Avodart) and tamsulosin, involved 5,000 men who took either one of the drugs alone, a combination pill containing both, or a placebo for four years. The men who took the combination pill experienced significantly decreased symptoms compared to all the others.

"The two medications joined forces in terms of symptom control," reported Claus Roehrborn, M.D., chairman of urology at University of Texas Southwestern Medical Center in Dallas. "On the strengths of both dutasteride and tamsulosin, participants reported fewer symptoms and we observed a 25 percent reduction in prostate volume."

The researchers found the combination drug reduced the need for surgery by 70 percent and decreased the risk of getting acute urinary retention by 65 percent compared to men who took tamsulosin alone. The combination drug proved to be only 19 percent more effective than dutasteride alone. Men taking the combination drug were less likely to discontinue therapy than the men taking either one alone.

As a result of the study, the U.S. Food and Drug Administration approved Jalyn, a single capsule containing 0.5 milligrams of dutasteride and 0.4 milligrams of tamsulosin, in June 2010.

The ideal candidate. Best for men with moderate to severe symptoms and a prostate 50 percent larger than normal.

Retrograde ejaculation

Retrograde, or dry, ejaculation means semen that is normally expelled from the urethra through the penis takes a U-turn and heads for the bladder. It is one of the most common side effects of all BPH treatments and can become permanent in about 10 percent of men who experience it.

Retrograde ejaculation does not pose a health threat but it does increase the risk of infertility.

Surgery — the 'simple' prostatectomy

Surgery is considered the treatment of last resort. It is recommended for men who have found no or little success from other treatments. Studies show improvement is greatest in men who experience the worst symptoms. Overall, marked improvement occurs in 93 percent of men with severe symptoms and 80 percent of men with moderate symptoms.

Surgery for BPH is called a simple prostatectomy and involves targeting and removing only the glandular tissue that is pressing up against the urethra. The word "simple," however, is a misnomer. From the patient's point of view it is anything but. It involves hospitalization, anesthesia, several days of catheterization, recovery time, and the risk of being among the small percentage that end up impotent and/or incontinent.

These are the procedures currently being used.

Transurethral resection prostatectomy (TURP)

TURP, which has been around for more than 20 years, is considered the gold standard for surgical BPH treatment, the one by which all other procedures are measured. More than 90 percent of BPH surgeries are performed by this method and it has the best success rate for men with urinary obstruction.

TURP involves removing the inner core of the prostate with a long, thin instrument called a resectoscope that is passed through the urethra and into the prostate. At the end of the resectoscope is an electrical wire loop that cuts away prostate tissue, piece by piece, and sends an electrical current of laser energy to seal blood vessels. As pieces of tissue are cut away, they are washed into the bladder and then flushed out of the body through the resectoscope.

At the end of the surgery, a catheter is inserted, which continually flushes fluid and monitors for bleeding in order to prevent blood clots. The catheter remains in place for up to three days. Some men report some pain and a great urgency to urinate for 12 to 24 hours after the surgery. Otherwise, there is little discomfort.

Studies show a marked improvement occurs in about 90 to 95 percent of men with severe symptoms and about 80 percent of men with moderate symptoms — a rate significantly better than what can be achieved with medication. Also, 95 percent of men who opt for TURP require no further treatment during the next five years.

The procedure takes about 45 minutes under general anesthesia and generally requires hospitalization for a day or two. In men with small prostates who are otherwise healthy, the procedure can be performed on an outpatient basis. Full recovery takes up to three weeks.

Advantages. Symptom relief is noticeable almost immediately and is greatest in men with the most severe symptoms. Generally, surgical procedures through catheters are much less risky than surgery through the abdominal wall.

Disadvantages. The surgery involves a lot of blood loss and transfusions may be necessary. Because the surgery is elective, you'll have the opportunity to bank your own blood prior to surgery.

Possible risks and complications. There is always a small, measurable risk of surgical problems or death as a consequence of surgery. Retrograde ejaculation is common. Approximately 5 to 10 percent of men experience impotence and 2 to 4 percent experience incontinence following surgery. Sexual dysfunction can be long-term.

The complication rate is 34 percent, according to one analysis. The most common complications are bleeding, urinary tract infection, and urinary retention. In rare instances, a man can develop TURP syndrome, a combination of difficult symptoms caused by the body absorbing too much of the water used to wash away excess prostate tissue. Symptoms include confusion, nausea, vomiting, high blood pressure, slow heart rate, and vision problems. The condition is treated with diuretics and goes away once the body's fluid and mineral balance is restored.

The ideal candidate. Appropriate for a man with severe lower urinary tract symptoms, including urinary obstruction.

Transurethral electrovaporization (TUVP)

This is a modified version of TURP. Instead of using a wire loop to cut away tissue, the resectoscope has a grooved roller at the end that delivers a powerful electric current to vaporize prostate tissue, which minimizes bleeding. Catheterization is also required after surgery.

An analysis of 20 studies found TUVP to be as effective as TURP in reducing prostate symptom scores and increasing peak urinary flow rates after one year.

Advantages. The main advantage is significantly less bleeding, so there is no need to bank blood. TUVP requires shorter catheterization time and shorter hospitalization than TURP. Generally, surgical procedures through catheters are much less risky than surgery through the abdominal wall.

Disadvantages. There is a greater risk of urinary retention and a greater chance that the surgery will have to be done again sometime in the future than there is with TURP.

Possible risks and complications. The same as for TURP, but slightly higher. There is always a small, measurable risk of surgical problems or death as a consequence of surgery.

The ideal candidate. Because the risk is low for retrograde ejaculation, this surgery is a better option for men concerned about fertility.

Surgery versus drugs

What's the more effective way to treat BPH — surgery or drugs?

According to a major 17-year-long community-based study conducted by the Mayo Clinic, transurethral resection of the prostate (TURP) proved to be the procedure that produced the best results. This was followed by laser vaporization surgery, alpha blocker medications, and androgen suppressant drugs.

"Patients who underwent TURP had the greatest decrease in both symptoms and incontinence compared to other treatment groups," reported Amy Krambeck, M.D., a Mayo Clinic urologist and the study's lead researcher. "Pre-TURP the incontinence rate was 64.5 percent and post-TURP it was 41.9 percent."

Overall, the study showed:

- urinary incontinence was common in all treatments despite an overall decrease in lower urinary tract symptoms.

- symptoms stabilized and did not get worse after all the treatments.

- surgery tended to be the choice in people with the worst symptoms.

Transurethral incision of the prostate (TUIP)

This procedure also uses a resectoscope, but instead of cutting away tissue, the surgeon makes two small incisions where the prostate meets the bladder with a powered knife or laser to relieve the pressure on the urethra. Studies show symptoms diminish an average of 73 percent in eight out of 10 men who have the procedure.

Advantages. The procedure takes less time and only requires an overnight stay in the hospital. Recovery is faster and the odds of complications are lower. TUIP has half the risk of causing retrograde ejaculation as TURP. Generally, surgical procedures through catheters are much less risky than surgery through the abdominal wall.

Disadvantages. TUIP has a lower success rate than TURP. A second surgery is required in 10 percent of men who have the operation.

Possible risks and complications. There is always a small, measurable risk of surgical problems or death as a consequence of surgery. The impotence risk is 4 to 25 percent. The risk of incontinence is 1 percent.

The ideal candidate. This surgery only benefits men with a small to medium-sized prostate, weighing no more than an ounce.

Open prostatectomy

This is the most invasive procedure and reserved for men who are not candidates for TURP or similar procedures. Like TURP it has a high success rate and almost always relieves symptoms. Some studies show it works better than TURP in relieving urinary blockage.

The operation requires making an incision below the navel and removing the inner portion of the prostate that surrounds the urethra. This is done in one of two ways. Suprapubic surgery involves opening the bladder and removing the tissue through the bladder. Retropubic involves moving the bladder aside and cutting directly into the prostate.

After suprapubic prostatectomy, two catheters are placed in the bladder, one through the urethra and the other through an incision made in the lower abdomen. They have to remain in place for three days to a week. In retropubic surgery, a catheter is placed in the bladder through the penis and urethra and remains for about a week. Hospital stay is from five to seven days and recovery takes from four to six weeks.

Advantages. It is the operation of choice when TURP is not possible. It involves less bleeding and has a faster recovery time.

Disadvantages. This procedure requires the longest hospitalization, catheterization, and recovery time. Surgery through the abdominal wall is generally much more risky than surgical procedures through catheters.

Possible risks and complications. There is always a small, measurable risk of surgical problems or death as a consequence of surgery. The risks and complications with this surgery are higher and more serious than with any other procedure. The most common complications are infection and excessive bleeding. Other serious complications, though rare, include pneumonia, heart attack, and pulmonary embolism, which is a blood clot that travels to the lungs. The risks of long-term impotence, incontinence, and retrograde ejaculation are also higher with this surgery than other procedures. The risk of impotence is 5 percent, but is higher in older men.

The ideal candidate. An otherwise healthy man with a prostate too large to undergo TURP is a good candidate for this procedure.

MIST opportunities

MIST, the acronym for minimally invasive surgical technique, is the hottest new line of therapy to treat an enlarged prostate — they literally zap tissue overgrowth with high-temperature heat, a procedure called thermoablation. There is an alphabet soup of procedures, based on the type of tool and energy used, and they go by names such as TUMT, TUNA, TEAP, and WIT, just to mention a few.

From the point of view of medicine and insurance companies, MISTs are the wave of the future because they are cost-efficient — no hospital time required — take less time, and carry a lower risk of side effects and complications. From the point of view of men with an enlarged prostate, MISTs offer the mother of all benefits — a stronger hold on your sexuality.

Studies to date show the benefits appear to be win-win: a significantly lower incidence of impotence and incontinence, a decreased risk of serious complications, a fast and painless recovery time and, of course, the major goal — relief from the bothersome symptoms of BPH that are close to, but not superior to, TURP. Or put another way, happier patients.

Still, in terms of scientific scrutiny, MISTs, for the most part, live in the research land of the great unknown, because the procedures generally are still considered new — some are still experimental — and research is limited. The biggest known downside is that having one of these procedures means it's likely that the symptoms of BPH will begin creeping back and eventually you will need to go through the same thing again. But to many guys, the greater security of sexual potency and continence is worth the tradeoff.

Several studies over the last few years have attempted to compare the strengths and weaknesses of different minimally invasive procedures to TURP. "The MISTs offer certain advantages over TURP," reported researchers from the University of Texas Medical School in Houston, who compared the outcomes of patients who had undergone four different MIST procedures to those who had TURP. "This must be tempered with the various shortcomings of the MISTs."

The advantages cited: better patient response to the surgery, fewer complications, quicker recovery, and the convenience and savings of shorter or no hospitalization. The shortcomings: higher rates of reoperations, lower urinary flow rates, and less established results.

Despite these limitations, the researchers concluded, general convenience and safety make "MISTs compelling alternatives to TURP for the surgical management of BPH."

Another limitation in your possible candidacy for a procedure could be your doctor. Not all urologists are trained in these procedures and some are difficult to master. If you have moderate or severe symptoms and your doctor recommends surgery, ask him about MIST and the pros and cons of each procedure. If he doesn't perform these procedures and doesn't know much about them, don't hesitate to ask for a referral to someone who does. It's in your best interest to check out all of your options, including MISTs, before deciding on the treatment that is best for you.

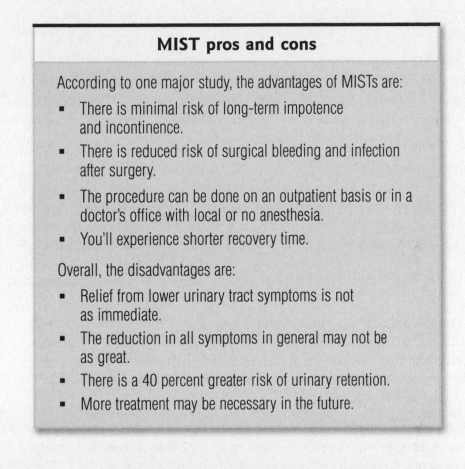

MIST pros and cons

According to one major study, the advantages of MISTs are:

- There is minimal risk of long-term impotence and incontinence.
- There is reduced risk of surgical bleeding and infection after surgery.
- The procedure can be done on an outpatient basis or in a doctor's office with local or no anesthesia.
- You'll experience shorter recovery time.

Overall, the disadvantages are:

- Relief from lower urinary tract symptoms is not as immediate.
- The reduction in all symptoms in general may not be as great.
- There is a 40 percent greater risk of urinary retention.
- More treatment may be necessary in the future.

MISTs come in several varieties. Though they are similar, each has its own unique approach. In a nutshell, here is what they are and what they accomplish.

Cooled thermo therapy

Formerly called transurethral microwave thermotherapy, this procedure is still called by its nickname TUMT. It is the MIST with the most scientific study behind it.

In this procedure, the surgeon guides a computer-controlled catheter that uses microwaves to heat and destroy excess prostate tissue. At the same time, it activates a cooling system to protect surrounding cells and the urethra from damage. The procedure requires catheterization from two days to two weeks after surgery. Antibiotics are generally prescribed to reduce the risk of infection from catheterization.

TUMT typically results in a 40 to 70 percent improvement in prostate symptom scores. In one five-year study comparing TUMT and TURP, researchers found no significant difference in their effect on improving symptoms or quality of life. However, 10 percent of the men who underwent TUMT required additional treatment compared to only 4 percent of men who underwent TURP.

Advantages. The procedure can be performed in a doctor's office or on an outpatient basis under no or local anesthesia. The risks of impotence and incontinence are very low. Generally, surgical procedures through catheters are much less risky than surgery through the abdominal wall.

Disadvantages. It can take from six weeks to three months to notice results.

Possible side effects and complications. Side effects include frequent urination, urgency, swelling of the urethra, discharge, and abdominal soreness that can last for a few weeks after treatment. There is always a small, measurable risk of surgical problems or death as a consequence of surgery.

The ideal candidate. Because of the device's design, it only can be used on men with medium-sized prostates, from 1 to 3 ounces, and moderate to severe symptoms.

Transurethral needle ablation (TUNA)

Unlike TUMT, which targets the entire prostate, TUNA aims for specific areas in the prostate. In this procedure, the surgeon inserts a rigid, telescopic catheter into the urethra and pushes tiny needles through it that emit radiofrequency energy to the targeted tissue. Catheterization is required for about five days following surgery.

Results are similar to TURP but risks are lower. In one study, reported in *The Journal of Urology*, the rate of impotence after surgery was 3 percent for men undergoing TUNA compared to 21 percent in men who received TURP. None of the men receiving TUNA therapy experienced retrograde ejaculation compared to 41 percent of men who underwent TURP. Less incontinence was reported in men who had TUNA therapy.

Advantages. There is a lower risk of sexual difficulties and incontinence. Generally, surgical procedures through catheters are much less risky than surgery through the abdominal wall.

Disadvantages. The procedure requires intravenous sedation in addition to local anesthesia.

Possible side effects and complications. There is always a small, measurable risk of surgical problems or death as a consequence of surgery.

The ideal candidate. Best for a man with a large prostate and urinary obstruction.

Photoselective vaporization of the prostate (PVP)

PVP "undoubtedly represents a change in care for surgical treatment of patients with lower urinary tract symptoms," proclaimed one European medical journal.

Also known as green light laser surgery, this procedure involves using a specially designed tool with a laser light that quickly vaporizes excess prostate tissue and seals the treated area with minimal bleeding. Studies show it can deliver immediate symptom relief and dramatic improvement in urinary flow rates similar to rates found with TURP.

The procedure takes from 10 to 30 minutes, depending on the size of the prostate, and is performed on an outpatient basis.

Advantages. Generally, surgical procedures through catheters are much less risky than surgery through the abdominal wall. In addition to offering immediate relief from symptoms, the procedure does not typically require catheterization afterwards and can be performed on an outpatient basis.

Disadvantages. The technique is difficult for doctors to learn. Full recovery can take several weeks.

Possible side effects and complications. This procedure has an overall low rate of side effects and complications, though retrograde ejaculation is common. However, there is always a small, measurable risk of surgical problems or death as a consequence of surgery. Blood in the urine is common after this procedure but generally does not require treatment.

The ideal candidate. Suitable for most men with moderate to severe symptoms.

Interstitial laser coagulation (ILC)

This procedure works the same way as TUNA, except that laser energy is used instead of radiofrequency energy to target specific prostate tissue. The tissue is heated, coagulated, and then destroyed. One study found symptom relief was about 10 percent lower than with TURP.

Advantages. Generally, surgical procedures through catheters are much less risky than surgery through the abdominal wall. There is a 30 percent lower risk of retrograde ejaculation than with TURP. One major study found the complication rate was less than 2 percent.

Disadvantages. Irritating urinary symptoms can persist for up to six weeks. There is also a high risk of needing a second procedure.

Possible risks and complications. This procedure has a low rate of risks and complications. The highest risk appears to be urinary tract infection. However, there is always a small, measurable risk of surgical problems or death as a consequence of surgery.

The ideal candidate. Best for a man with a medium-size prostate who does not have a urinary obstruction.

Water-induced thermotherapy (WIT)

This therapy uses temperature-controlled heated water to destroy excess prostate tissue. In the procedure, a surgeon uses a catheter containing multiple shafts to insert a balloon in the middle of the prostate. Water flows into the balloon to heat targeted prostate tissue. The destroyed tissue either escapes through the urethra or is reabsorbed by the body.

Advantages. There are no adverse effects on sexual function. It can help relieve problems in men with sexual dysfunction prior to having the procedure. Generally, surgical procedures through catheters are much less risky than surgery through the abdominal wall.

Disadvantages. It can take up to three months to feel noticeable effects and up to a year to achieve maximum symptom relief.

Possible risks and complications. There are few risks and complications associated with this procedure. However, there is always a small, measurable risk of surgical problems or death as a consequence of surgery.

The ideal candidate. Good for a man with moderate to severe symptoms of urinary obstruction.

Stents

In this procedure a surgeon uses a catheter to insert a plastic or metal expandable device into the urethra to keep the passage open. It is used when quick action is required to relieve urinary retention.

Advantages. Generally, surgical procedures through catheters are much less risky than surgery through the abdominal wall. The catheter can be inserted quickly under spinal anesthesia, catheterization is not required, and recovery is quick.

Disadvantages. It can cause annoying urinary symptoms, such as urgency and frequent and painful urination, for days or weeks after the procedure.

Risks and possible complications. There is a possibility of bladder stones forming around the stent. There is little known about long-term risks or complications. However, there is always a small, measurable risk of surgical problems or death as a consequence of surgery. It may be wise to avoid this procedure until more is known about long-term results.

The ideal candidate. This procedure is reserved for older men with acute urinary retention who are in poor overall health.

Prostatitis: when infection sets in

Prostatitis is not one, but a cluster of afflictions that share a common bond in the men it strikes — pain and discomfort. It can be easy to treat or tough to treat. The symptoms can disappear almost overnight or linger like in-laws on a summer vacation. How menacing it is and how long it will hang around really depends on the type of prostatitis you have.

Prostatitis is either acute, meaning it brings on pain and discomfort that lasts a few days, or chronic, meaning the symptoms come and go, and then come back again. It can be bacterial, meaning it's caused by a specific organism, or it can be nonbacterial, meaning it's caused by something other than bacteria — but what is still a medical mystery.

These types of prostatitis have one thing in common — infection that produces pain in the pelvic region, urination problems, difficulties having sex, and an overall malaise. The most distinguishable symptom is pain in the perineum, the area between the anus and the base of the penis, especially when sitting. Some men say it feels like they're sitting on a golf ball. Pain can also show up in the lower back, groin, penis, testicles, or scrotum.

Bacterial prostatitis may sound like the most sinister type, but it's not because there's a simple test to confirm it and it's usually easy to treat. Nonbacterial prostatitis, however, is a complex and confounding condition that is often hard to identify. There is no standard diagnostic test to confirm it and no "best" way to treat it. This leaves a lot of guys in a very painful predicament because it is by far the most common form of prostatitis. An estimated 40 percent of visits to a urologist's office are for pain that turns out to be chronic nonbacterial prostatitis. The disease can strike at any age, but the typical guy plagued by its relentless symptoms is in his 40s.

Prostatitis 4 ways

The National Institutes of Health recognizes four distinct types of prostatitis.

Nonbacterial or abacterial. The most common and hardest to treat, it is also called chronic prostatitis/chronic pelvic pain syndrome that you may see as the acronym CP/CPPS. It can be inflammatory or noninflammatory. Its cause is unknown.

Acute bacterial. The least common and easiest to treat, it is caused by infectious organisms.

Chronic bacterial. Defined by symptoms that last at least three months, it's usually caused by repeated urinary tract infections.

Asymptomatic inflammatory prostatitis. This type has no symptoms and is usually discovered through an evaluation for another illness or blood work that reveals an increased level of white blood cells, which is a sign of inflammation.

Nonbacterial prostatitis

So exactly what is chronic nonbacterial prostatitis? The National Institutes of Health sums it up this way: "Chronic abacterial prostatitis is a common, bothersome syndrome in men, which is poorly defined, poorly understood, and poorly treated."

For sure. A lot of doctors aren't even familiar with it. A recent survey of primary care physicians throughout the United States — and more than half of them were men — found that 16 percent were "not at all familiar" with prostatitis and 48 percent were "not at all familiar" with the different classifications. The disease is so misunderstood that its symptoms lead many doctors to mistakenly diagnose it as benign prostatic hyperplasia (BPH).

Thousands of studies have been conducted on prostatitis, but finding a cause still eludes researchers. Some experts believe the condition is caused by bacteria that are yet to be identified. Others believe it is not a prostate problem at all, but flare-ups caused by spasms in pelvic muscles. Another theory says it is an autoimmune disease in which the immune system mistakenly attacks healthy prostate tissue and causes inflammation. Many possible causes have been examined over the years, though there is no conclusive evidence on what could be the causes. Some of the major suspects are:

- bladder infection
- caffeine
- catheterization
- dehydration
- infrequent ejaculation
- unprotected sex
- stress
- swimming in polluted water
- chronic urinary problems
- vasectomy
- zinc deficiency

"Considering the high prevalence of symptoms attributed to prostatitis and the many studies conducted during the past 50 years that have attempted to define its causes and optimal treatments, it is surprising how little we know about this syndrome," says Benjamin A. Lipsky, M.D., an infectious disease specialist and professor of medicine at University of Washington Medical School.

Do you have prostatitis?

The National Institutes of Health (NIH) developed this question-naire, called the Chronic Prostatitis Symptom Index (NIH-CPSI) in 2002 to help doctors evaluate the impact of symptoms on the lives of men with chronic nonbacterial prostatitis. You can use it, too. For your answers, use the numeric value in the parentheses.

Pain or discomfort

1. In the last week, have you experienced any pain or discomfort in the following areas:

   Area between the rectum and testicles (perineum):
   ☐ Yes (1) ☐ No (0)

   Testicles:
   ☐ Yes (1) ☐ No (0)

   Tip of the penis, unrelated to urination:
   ☐ Yes (1) ☐ No (0)

   Below the waist in the pubic or bladder area:
   ☐ Yes (1) ☐ No (0)

2. In the last week, have you experienced:

   Pain or burning during urination?
   ☐ Yes (1) ☐ No (0)

   Pain or discomfort during or after ejaculation?
   ☐ Yes (1) ☐ No (0)

3. How often have you had pain or discomfort in any of these areas over the last week?

   ☐ Never (0)   ☐ Rarely (1)   ☐ Sometimes (2)

   ☐ Often (3)   ☐ Usually (4)   ☐ Always (5)

4. On a scale of 0 to 10, which number best describes your average pain or discomfort on the days that you had it over the last week?

										Pain as bad as you can imagine
   No pain
   0   1   2   3   4   5   6   7   8   9   10

A. Total pain score: _____

Urination

5. How often during the last week have you had a sensation of not emptying your bladder completely after you finished urinating?

- ☐ Not at all (0)
- ☐ Less than 1 time in 5 (1)
- ☐ Less than half the time (2)
- ☐ About half the time (3)
- ☐ More than half the time (4)
- ☐ Almost always (5)

6. How often during the last week have you had to go again less than 2 hours after you had finished urinating?

- ☐ Not at all (0)
- ☐ Less than 1 time in 5 (1)
- ☐ Less than half the time (2)
- ☐ About half the time (3)
- ☐ More than half the time (4)
- ☐ Almost always (5)

B. Total urinary symptoms score: _____

Impact of symptoms/quality of life

7. During the last week, how much have your symptoms kept you from doing the kinds of things you would usually do?

- ☐ None (0)
- ☐ Only a little (1)
- ☐ Some (2)
- ☐ A lot (3)

8. How much did you think about your symptoms during the last week?

- ☐ None (0)
- ☐ Only a little (1)
- ☐ Some (2)
- ☐ A lot (3)

9. If you were to spend the rest of your life with your symptoms just the way they have been during the last week, how would you feel about it?

☐ Delighted (0)   ☐ Pleased (1)   ☐ Mostly satisfied (2)

☐ Mixed (3)   ☐ Mostly dissatisfied (4)

☐ Unhappy (5)   ☐ Terrible (6)

C. *Total quality of life impact score* _____

To determine your Symptoms Scale Score, add *A* and *B*   _____

To determine your Total Score and the degree of your   _____
prostatitis, add *A* through *C*

What your scores mean

A Symptoms Scale Score of 1-9 means your symptoms are mild; 10-18 means they are moderate; and 19-31 means they are severe.

A Total Score of 1-14 means you have mild prostatitis; 15-29 means the disease is moderate; and 30-43 indicates it is severe.

Any treatment you try that drops your score 4 to 6 points means you are making significant improvement.

Though the cause of this condition is a mystery, the impact it has on a man's quality of life is not. Bacterial prostatitis can leave a guy in misery. Its symptoms can be relentless, lasting for several weeks and then go away, only to come back again. In addition to the pain and urinary problems, it messes with your love life. Some men complain about painful ejaculation. Others say ejaculating helps relieve pain. The syndrome of symptoms can cause such anguish that it leaves many men depressed and in psychological pain. One study found it can be as life-altering as having a heart attack or diabetes.

Trying out treatments

The main reason why nonbacterial prostatitis is so miserable to live with is because there is no therapy that has been found to measurably help relieve the symptoms. Thousands of studies have investigated dozens of potential remedies and nothing comes out the full-court advantage. What helps some men doesn't work at all for others. Most often, a single therapy only offers minimal to modest symptom relief. What appears to help best, according to new research, is combining two or more of the therapies that have been found to produce results in some men some of the time. These are among the therapies that have shown to have a positive effect on their own in reducing symptoms in some men.

Try antibiotics first — and only once. Most men with chronic, painful prostatitis don't test positive for a bacterial infection, but doctors frequently prescribe antibiotics "just in case." In fact, a study involving more than 23,000 men with nonbacterial prostatitis found that most of them were prescribed antibiotics, according to *The American Journal of Medicine*.

Antibiotics are appropriate for some men but not for others, says J. Curtis Nickel, M.D., a urologist and infectious disease expert at Queens University and Kingston General Hospital in Canada who examined all the current therapies being used to treat prostatitis. He found that antibiotics seem to only help men who have recently been afflicted with the disease or have had symptoms for a relatively short time. On average, 75 percent of these men found relief after taking ciprofloxacin (Cipro), which belongs to a strong class of drugs called fluoroquinolones that are used for hard-to-fight infections. However, only 20 to 30 percent of men with long-standing symptoms responded to the same drug therapy. Even with all their strength, fluoroquinolones do not appear to be powerful enough to combat long-standing inflammation.

Dr. Nickel cautions against taking antibiotics for too long, especially if they aren't doing you much good, because you can build a resistance to them.

Give antibiotics a boost. Ask your doctor about the immune-suppressing steroid prednisone (Deltasone). Preliminary research in China found that combining prednisone with fluoroquinolone effectively relieved pain and urinary problems and increased overall quality of life in men after just four weeks of treatment.

Ask about alpha blockers for urinary symptom relief. Some studies show that alpha blockers, which were designed to bring urinary tract relief for men with BPH, can offer "modest" relief from prostatitis. As with antibiotics, they only appear to benefit newly diagnosed men. "Alpha blockers cannot be recommended for men with long-standing symptoms who have tried and failed alpha blockers in the past," says Dr. Nickel. The alpha blockers Dr. Nickel found that help offer relief are alfuzosin, tamsulosin, and terazosin.

Give anti-inflammatories a try. Some doctors recommend taking over-the-counter anti-inflammatory drugs, such as ibuprofen (Advil, Motrin) and naproxen (Aleve), for pain relief.

Get out of your funk. Depression is a common side effect to living with the pain and other limitations of prostatitis. If you're depressed, tell your doctor. There is a relationship between physical and mental pain, and one can affect the other. Depression can make pain feel worse than it really is. Some men have been pleasantly surprised to find that pain didn't feel as severe when they were taking antidepressants. Studies have found an association between depression and symptom relief from these antidepressant medications: citalopram (Celexa), duloxetin (Cymbalta), and nortriptyline (Aventyl).

Go natural. Several studies report that men with prostatitis have found relief from taking the herbal extracts bee pollen and saw palmetto and the antioxidant quercetin. As with prescription medications, the sooner you try them after the onset of symptoms, the better. You can find out more information about these individual substances in Chapter 11.

Think yourself well with biofeedback. This technique employs special instrumentation that teaches you how to recognize involuntary physiological changes in your body, such as your heart rate and blood pressure, and how to use your mind to control them. Biofeedback for prostate diseases concentrates on learning how to control pelvic floor muscles for urinary control. Pelvic floor biofeedback dates back 30 years. Recent studies show that it can produce satisfactory short-term effects.

Biofeedback requires special equipment in which electrodes are attached to the skin so you can observe the involuntary movements of the pelvic floor on a monitor. A trained biofeedback specialist teaches you how to sense these involuntary actions and react to them. Your doctor and the Internet can help get you on the track to find the therapy in your vicinity.

Count on TENS. Transcutaneous electrical nerve stimulation (TENS) employs high-frequency electrical current to release pain. In the procedure a technician attaches gelled pads to the skin of the perineum, which sends pulsed waves of electrical stimulations to the peripheral nerve fibers. In one study, 24 patients who received the treatment along with antibiotics five times a week for four weeks experienced significantly more pain relief than men taking antibiotics alone and men taking antibiotics plus analgesics.

Press the trigger. The American Urological Association (AUA) reports that men have found pain relief through a type of muscle massage called myofascial trigger point therapy, which is based on the belief that pain in one location can be released by manipulating trigger points residing elsewhere in the body. Though the mechanism of pain in prostatitis is not fully understood, there is evidence indicating it emanates from a chronically contracted pelvic floor. Using a technique called pelvic trigger point release, the contraction is broken by manipulating trigger points in the muscles of the arms, back, and rectum.

The AUA tested this theory on 125 men who enrolled in a six-day "prostate boot camp" where they learned about myofascial trigger point release and relaxation. The men had been living with the pain of prostatitis for an average of eight years. After seven months of therapy, 68 percent of them experienced a significant 6-point drop on the NIH Chronic Prostate Symptom Index.

You can find a therapist near you by searching the website *www.myofascialtherapy.org*.

Let someone needle you. Pricking the skin with tiny thin needles in strategic locations on the body is the point of the ancient Chinese healing art of acupuncture. According to traditional Chinese medicine, acupuncture restores vital energy, called *Qi*, along meridians that lead to specific organs.

In one of several studies, acupuncture proved to be 25 percent more effective than antibiotic therapy in reducing symptoms scores in men with prostatitis. In another study, reported in the journal *Pain Medicine*, men reported a 50 percent decrease in their NIH-CPSI scores after getting acupuncture treatments for six weeks.

Acupuncture is a painless procedure and is relaxing. Some people fall asleep while having it done. Make sure you go to someone who is a certified acupuncturist. You can get help finding one near you through the National Certification Commission for Acupuncture and Oriental Medicine website at *www.nccaom.org*.

Take your prostate global. What feels good on the outside is also good for what's inside — and that includes the pain generated by an inflamed prostate. One study, reported in *The Journal of Urology*, found that a full-body therapeutic massage for one hour a week for 10 weeks resulted in an average 7.6 drop in the Chronic Prostate Symptom Index for all 48 men who had enrolled in the study. The men, who were all in their early-to-mid 40s, had been experiencing symptoms for three years.

Rub your prostate the right way. One of the best things you can do for your ailing prostate is to give it a personal massage. Prostate massage is excellent therapy, because it helps drain glandular secretions and promotes an increase in blood flow. But don't let the word massage mislead you. It can be more than a tad uncomfortable. You know how it felt when your doctor just touched your inflamed prostate. Massaging it will generate the same feeling, but for longer. Think of it as good pain, the kind that will help make you feel a whole lot better in the long run. You can help alleviate the pain and discomfort by taking ibuprofen about an hour beforehand. Taking a hot bath before the massage is also helpful.

You can do the massage yourself or enlist the help of a trained medical technician or even a spouse. It's a good idea to have your doctor demonstrate the technique for you before doing it at home.

How to do a prostate massage

Ready the equipment:

- a pair of latex gloves
- KY lubricating jelly
- paper towels for discharge from penis

First, check with your doctor to see if she agrees that you are a good candidate for self-administration of this procedure.

Lie down on your side and bring your hand around your back. This is better than reaching your rectum by putting your hands through your legs. Gently insert a lubricated gloved finger into your rectum. About an inch and a half in, you'll feel a bump. This is your prostate. If may feel bigger than you imagined because it's swollen. Generally, you can feel a depression in the middle. This is the starting point for the massage, though if the gland is too swollen you may not detect it.

Firmly rub the prostate from side to side using slow, continuous pressure. You'll know you're doing it right if you feel a slight stinging or burning.

Exercise gently. Exercising is hard when you're in pain and some men say it is darn near impossible. Instead of jogging or doing other exercise that pounds the prostate, go for gentle exercise. Dozens of studies show that gentle exercise that employs mind-body control, such as yoga and tai chi, can help alleviate the tenderness and fatigue associated with chronic painful disease. While no studies have been conducted on these exercises and prostatitis, many doctors recommend them as an alternative to more strenuous exercises.

Get out of the saddle. The kind of exercise you don't want to do is one that is hard on the perineum, which is the point of so much pain. This means no prolonged bicycle or horseback riding. Too much time in the saddle compresses the perineum, which starves the urethra, bladder, and prostate of blood.

Put your prostate on ice. Putting an ice pack up against your bottom can help reduce pain and inflammation. Even better, apply it directly to your prostate, like you would a suppository. Place an ice cube in water until the rough edges melt, then insert it into the rectum. Doctors report that it can give you hours of relief.

Avoid getting constipated. Hard bowel movements can put painful pressure on the prostate. Eating fiber-rich foods can keep your bowels moving easily. If you generally don't eat a lot of fiber, add it to your diet slowly. Adding too much too quickly can cause irregularity. You should be getting 35 grams a day of fiber to keep your plumbing humming. Good sources include whole grains, beans, fruits, and vegetables. You should also drink plenty of water because it helps get your bowels in motion.

Keep yourself well-watered. It would seem that drinking less water so you don't have to urinate so much is the sensible approach, but it turns out that the opposite is true. You need plenty of water in your system to keep your urine from becoming too concentrated, which could cause a bladder infection. Get at least eight glasses a day.

As a last resort, surgery is an option — but: Having surgery as a means to beat prostatitis is controversial. Those in the pro-surgery camp point to studies showing that a minimally invasive surgical technique used to treat BPH called transurethral microwave thermotherapy (TUMT) can be a "safe, effective, and long-lasting alternative to other treatments" for prostatitis. However, opponents caution that the benefits are not great enough to outweigh the risks for most people. The technique involves sending computer-regulated microwave heat through a catheter to destroy excess tissue on selected sites in the prostate. To find out more about it, see page 65.

Diagnosing prostatitis

If you're experiencing any of the symptoms of prostatitis, your first line of defense is to see a specialist who is up on the latest research and therapy for prostate problems, and prostatitis in particular. That would be a urologist. As a survey conducted by the Chronic Prostatitis Collaborative Research Network shows, primary care physicians generally do not have a lot of experience in managing the illness. Only 62 percent of the physicians polled reported ever seeing a patient with the symptoms of nonbacterial prostatitis.

When you see a urologist, he will perform a digital rectal exam to feel the prostate. Though this test is typically uncomfortable, touching an inflamed prostate can be downright painful. If the prostate feels squishy and you wince, it pretty much tells the doctor what he's dealing with.

Most likely, he will order these tests:

- **Blood panel.** This is a simple test in which blood is drawn to check for the level of white blood cells. If the count is high, it is a sign of infection.

- **Urinalysis.** This is the pee-in-the-cup test that can determine the presence of infection. The lab tests your urine by using a chemically treated dipstick. The strip will turn different colors depending on what's in your urine.

- **Urine culture.** This test, also called the Meares-Stamey four-cup test, helps detect and identify the presence of bacteria. It involves giving four urine samples in sequence while in the doctor's office. In cup number one, you release enough urine to cover the bottom of the cup. In the second cup, called the midstream sample, you urinate a little more, but do not release it all. Before you urinate into the third cup, the doctor will massage the prostate. This stimulates the penis to expel a few drops of secretions from the gland. It goes in cup number three. If nothing comes out, the secretions will show up when you finish urinating into cup number four.

Bacterial prostatitis

Acute bacterial prostatitis is rare. It comes on so quickly and so painfully that a doctor is the only person you want to see. That's good, because immediate attention is just what it needs.

For all the pain and worry it creates, the condition is easy to diagnose and treat. A digital rectal exam and a urinalysis or urine culture are generally all that are needed to confirm it. If you've recently had a new sexual encounter, your doctor might also order a test to detect chlamydia or gonorrhea, common sexually transmitted diseases.

The good news is that antibiotics can relieve the symptoms almost as quickly as they came on and more than likely they will never come back. You need to stay on the medication for the full term of treatment, which could be as long as four or six weeks. Either a broad-spectrum penicillin, such as piperacillin (Pipracit) or cephalosporin (Ceclor) should do the trick.

Acute bacterial prostatitis is rare and accounts for less than 1 percent of prostatitis cases. Fifty to 80 percent of cases are caused by a strain of *E. coli*, the prevalent bacteria we generally associate with food poisoning. It also can be caused by infected urine or a sexually transmitted disease. Sometimes it can turn up as a complication of a rectal prostate biopsy.

Symptoms of acute bacterial infection are:

■ fever, chills, and other flu-like symptoms

■ pain in the lower back and perineum, the area between the scrotum and anus

■ painful and/or urgent urination

■ a weak urinary stream

Chronic bacterial prostatitis feels like an acute case that doesn't want to go away. In fact, the condition isn't considered chronic until symptoms have persisted for three months!

The number one cause of the infrequent cases of chronic bacterial prostatitis is repeated urinary tract infections. Sometimes an acute case that doesn't respond to antibiotics can lead to a chronic condition, but this is rarely the case. In fact, unless you've had a run of urinary tract infections, your chance of getting this chronic condition is slim. In rare instances, prostate stones that harbor bacteria can lead to chronic infection.

Bacterial prostatitis is chronic because the infection is highly resistant to antibiotics. The prostate isn't fighting off the infection because the ducts have become blocked with inflamed debris. The prostate has a limited blood supply, making it difficult for your immune system to properly defend your prostate from invaders. The poor blood supply makes it difficult for antibiotics to reach the prostate.

"Treating chronic bacterial prostatitis requires prolonged therapy with an antibiotic that penetrates the prostate," says Dr. Benjamin Lipsky, an infectious disease specialist and professor of medicine at University of Washington Medical School. The recommended treatment is stronger and longer antibiotic therapy with fluoroquinolone.

The symptoms of chronic bacterial prostatitis are:

- frequent urinary urgency
- painful urination
- a feeling of heaviness or pressure behind the scrotum
- pelvic pain and/or pain in the lower back or lower section of the stomach
- painful ejaculation
- symptoms that come and go

In addition to taking the antibiotics, you can help speed your recovery with these self-help tactics.

Ask about other drugs. Ask your doctor about muscle-relaxing drugs, such as alpha blockers. They can help relieve the bladder, pelvic, and rectal muscle spasms that contribute to pain.

Lay off the stimulants. This means no alcohol or caffeine. They can irritate the prostate and trigger spasms that cause urine to backwash into your prostate, irritating it further.

Get the spice out of your life. Spicy foods, chocolate, and tomato products can do the same.

Sit up. An infected prostate is so painful it can make sitting just about unbearable. Try sitting on a doughnut-shaped cushion that is made to ease the discomfort of hemorrhoids. You should be able to find one in a drugstore. Also, men report sitting on a hard chair rather than an easy chair is much easier on the pain.

Go soak for a while. Submerging your bottom in a tub of warm water for 15 minutes several times a day will help improve blood circulation in your prostate and help speed healing.

Get lots of sex. Yes, pain sometimes has its rewards. Some experts believe that regular ejaculation helps ease an infection because it routinely empties the glands and ducts of the prostate, releasing its hold on infection.

A little Botox, anyone?

Would you let someone inject a little poison directly into your prostate in the name of science? Thousands of men have so far and they got what they were hoping for — relief from the urinary problems caused by prostate disease.

Botox, which comes from botulinum toxin type A, is best known as an anti-aging agent to erase facial wrinkles. For the last several years, studies in the United States and Asia have been investigating it for its potential in helping ease the discomfort associated with prostatitis and an enlarged prostate. To date, Botox injections have been found to offer men significant improvement in urinary functions that can last up to a year. In one study, 80 percent of the men with urinary obstruction found they could completely empty their bladder.

It's not clear exactly how Botox works, but it appears to weaken certain muscles and block certain nerves involved with involuntary urinary regulation.

Doctors fall short of recommending it as a remedy for prostate disease as it is still in the experimental stage.

Prostate stones: blocked ducts

You've heard of kidney stones and gallstones. But, prostate stones? You bet. And even if you've never heard of them, there is a chance that you could have them. You just don't know it.

Unlike kidney or urinary stones, which are extremely painful and must be treated to prevent damage to the organ, prostate stones are benign and, for the most part, painless.

Stones form in the prostate when prostatic secretion can't escape the gland because the ducts are blocked. They eventually dry out and calcify. This can happen in men with an enlarged prostate or prostatitis.

There really isn't anything that needs to be done if you have prostate stones, as long as they aren't causing you any discomfort. You could have them for years and not know it. Most often they are discovered by accident through an examination for another condition.

Prostate stones eventually dissolve on their own. Sometimes, though, stones can get large and start causing urinary trouble similar to an enlarged prostate. The main distinction is that you'll feel muscle cramps in the pelvis and lower stomach and possibly lower back pain.

If you are having these symptoms, see your doctor for treatment. There is currently no medication to treat prostate stones. The only remedy is to remove them surgically.

When the doctor says it's cancer

If you've been diagnosed with prostate cancer or your doctor suspects you have prostate cancer, take a deep breath and get a grip on your emotions. Though there is nothing good about a diagnosis of cancer, there is some good news when the diagnosis is prostate cancer.

Prostate cancer is the horse and buggy of cancers — it usually advances slowly. It is so slow-growing, in fact, that virtually any man who lives long enough will develop some degree of prostate cancer — but he'll usually die of something else. The majority of men diagnosed with prostate cancer — an estimated 220,000 a year — have early-stage cancer, meaning it's likely that it could take years before the disease is threatening enough to treat, and it's quite possible it may never need to be treated.

The reason for this is twofold. One, is the way the cancer grows. At this very moment, millions of healthy cells in your body are dying and being replaced by new ones. The rate at which cells replicate varies from organ to organ and tissue to tissue. Sometimes, however, a cell experiences a random mutation during normal cell division. Some are lethal to the cell; some are not. Or the cell gets damaged, perhaps by an inherited defect, radiation, or a toxic invader. Then, instead of dying to make way for a stronger healthy cell, it may mutate — it divides and multiplies. One cell becomes two, two become four, four become eight. How long it takes for cells to multiply in this way is called doubling time. Eventually, these mutant cells may gang up and cluster into a tumor. The verdict is binding: You have cancer. In the prostate this process moves slower than it does in other organs. Science shows that most cancers have doubling times measured in weeks. Prostate cancer cell doubling time can be measured in months and even years.

The second reason prostate cancer may not pose a threat is the fact it is so easily diagnosed. Largely due to PSA testing, prostate cancer cells can be discovered at a very early stage, often before a lump could possibly be detected on a manual physical exam and long before they pose any kind of threat. In fact, some doctors argue that early prostate cancer should be called something other than cancer — just as cancerous changes in skin cells are sometimes referred to as "precancer."

This is where the controversy of PSA testing comes in. Rising PSA levels most frequently lead to biopsy, biopsy leads to early detection, and early detection leads to aggressive treatment. Because the prostate is so small, biopsy is insidiously accurate. Even the tiniest nonthreatening cancer cells may show up in a random sampling. As you read in Part 1, it's the major reason why the top experts agree that prostate cancer today is overdiagnosed and overtreated.

Knowing this may actually be raising your anxiety because it leaves you wondering: *Whom do you trust*? You can assuage your fear and find security in who you're putting in charge of your care by understanding the facts about your disease and its diagnosis and not rushing into any treatment until you are able to make an informed and unemotional decision.

Mark Scholz, M.D., an oncologist who specializes in prostate cancer and author of *Invasion of the Prostate Snatchers*, sums it up succinctly: "Realistically, the PSA itself is not the problem. The problem is doctors and patients overreacting to the information PSA supplies."

So before you overreact, let's get a handle on your disease, starting with the question everyone seems to want answered.

Why me?

The simple answer to that question is: nobody knows. Prostate cancer is among the many cancers still baffling researchers. As with most other cancers, scientists have yet to come up with a reason why one man will be diagnosed at age 50 and another at age 80, while yet another may never appear to be in jeopardy. They suspect, though, that it is not just one factor but rather a confluence of several dynamics, both environmental and genetic, that come together like the perfect storm.

While many of them are probably still unknown, science has identified a handful of traits, or risk factors, that increase the likelihood that certain men will get a diagnosis of the disease. They fall into good news/bad news categories. Let's start with the bad news — the risks you can't do a thing about.

Family history. Studies of identical and fraternal twins reveal a strong hereditary link. Your risk rises with the number of first-degree relatives, meaning a brother or your father, who had the disease. It also rises if you've had any relative who was diagnosed with prostate cancer before age 60.

Hereditary prostate cancer is transmitted from father to son and from father to daughter and then to her son.

Recent genetic studies suggest that 5 to 10 percent of prostate cancer has a hereditary link. Nearly half of men with a hereditary link develop the cancer before age 55.

Age. The longer you live, the more likely you are to be diagnosed with the disease. The risk of being diagnosed with prostate cancer rises dramatically with age, more so than with any other type of cancer. The disease can occur at any age, but it is most often found in men older than 50. More than 75 percent of tumors are found in men age 65 and older.

Race. Any man can get prostate cancer, but black men are nearly twice as likely to get prostate cancer as white men and they are at greater risk for getting a more aggressive form of the disease. Incidence in the United States is lowest among Asians. This is another factor that suggests a genetic link, although environmental factors such as differing blood levels of vitamin D also may play a role.

Living in the United States. The United States by far leads the world in both the incidence of prostate disease and death from the disease, though the death rate is starting to decline. In fact, it is second only to lung cancer as the leading cancer threat to American men.

Part of the reason for the high incidence of diagnosis and the low death rate is early detection through PSA screening, making it a double-edged sword. However, American men reigned supreme even before the PSA test. The reason leads to flipping the coin to the good news — good because they are all things we can do something about.

Living *la vida loca*. Or to translate Ricky Martin's Latin music hit, living the crazy life. The American lifestyle is intrinsically connected to prostate cancer, as it is with many other cancers. There is growing evidence that 90 percent of the blame for the high rate of prostate disease in American men can be pointed directly to the typical Western lifestyle.

Too much food in general and fat in particular increase your risk of getting the disease. So does not eating enough vegetables, snubbing fish for dinner, never seeing the inside of a gym, and having a belly that resembles a beach ball — all things you can do something about. In fact, there are so many simple but meaningful adjustments you can make in your lifestyle that are beneficial to your prostate, they fill up a third of this book. You can find them in Part 3.

There is even evidence that you can manipulate your genetic predisposition to the disease. A relatively new science called epigenetics has demonstrated that even if you have a gene that puts you at risk for the cancer, it does not mean that your body will activate that gene. Environmental factors — such as exposure to toxins, poor diet, and lifestyle choices — and even aging itself can determine if the gene stays dormant or rears its nasty disposition.

Vasectomy: is there a link?

Not proven, but scientists fall short of saying unequivocally that there is no link between vasectomy and an increased risk of prostate cancer.

An association between the two was first noted in 1993 when a pair of studies involving 77,000 men, reported in the *Journal of the American Medical Association*, found that having a vasectomy increased a man's risk of prostate cancer by more than 50 percent.

Since then, however, other studies involving much smaller groups of men couldn't find any link at all.

The official word from the National Cancer Institute: If there is a link, it is "very weak, at best."

Testosterone: fueling cancer

Though the cause of prostate cancer still eludes scientists, they do know what makes it grow: the male hormone testosterone.

Testosterone, of course, is hardly a bad thing. It's what makes a man a man and, well, manly. The prostate gland is exquisitely sensitive to the presence and absence of testosterone. Testosterone is what transformed you from a gangly teenager to a virile man. It influences your persona — your self-esteem, your frame of mind, your energy, and your lust for life and love. It determines the sound of your voice, your height, your muscle mass, the size of your libido, and the quality of your erections. It can also make prostate cancer grow.

It is not fully understood how testosterone fuels prostate cancer and to what degree, but there is no doubt that it can make cancer grow. How fast, however, isn't known. Sometimes the growth rate is so slow that many doctors question the rationale of resorting to aggressive treatments — those designed to stop the production or activation of testosterone but which can also threaten a man's quality of life.

Prostate cancer can also grow independent of testosterone and other hormones but how this occurs is also not fully understood. What is known is that prostate cancer, like all cancers, is an opportunist. It takes advantage of compromised and impaired immunity, a bad diet, a sluggish body, and certain genes to set up a life of its own and throw your life off course.

'Normal' age-specific PSA

The prostate enlarges with age and an enlarged prostate makes PSA levels go up, so it only seems logical to expect normal levels to creep up as you get older. Though some experts say that there is no such thing as "normal" when it comes to PSA, there is a school of thought that believes that normal should be adjusted according to age and race as follows:

Age	Black	White	Asian
40-49	2.0	2.5	2.0
50-59	4.0	3.5	3.0
60-69	4.5	4.5	4.0
70-79	5.5	6.5	5.0

Source: Mayo Clinic Proceedings 1997

How prostate cancer spreads

At some point, if there is enough growth and if they are left untreated, prostate cancer cells may break away from the mass and enter the bloodstream to prowl around for another part of the body to invade. If these mobile cells should take root in another place, this migration is called metastasis, meaning "change of state." In other words, the cancer has spread.

Most cancer cells that become mobile often target a vital organ for a new lodging place, such as the lungs, liver, or the brain. This spreading gets you precariously close to death in a short time.

Prostate cancer works a little differently. It appears to always follow the same *modus operandi* when it spreads. It makes its way to the seminal vesicles, small tubular glands that secrete part of the fluid that makes semen. These glands sit above the prostate and behind the bladder. From here it spreads to the lymph nodes and then the bones. This is when prostate cancer becomes life-threatening. However, it is a slow process.

For example, when other types of cancer start to spread, survival is often counted in months and at most usually a few years. Studies show that it typically takes 13 years, or longer, for those cases of prostate cancer that eventually spread to advance to the point where they are life-threatening. This is why doctors now consider it pointless for men in their 70s with normal PSA levels to continue to get screenings for prostate cancer. It's very likely they will die of other causes before prostate cancer might become a problem.

Signs and symptoms

A bad side of prostate cancer is that it leaves no calling card. For most men, the first indication that they may have the disease comes when a PSA screening shows the level jumped since the last test a year ago. This is the major issue with PSA testing because it is not a true biomarker for cancer, meaning that it cannot detect the presence of cancer cells. An elevated PSA is only a warning sign that something abnormal is happening in the prostate. Any prostate disease or problem will elevate PSA.

Prostate cancer only starts to give warning signs as it begins to advance. Symptoms start to appear in your urinary canal. Frequent, slow, or painful urination, problems getting an erection, and pain in and around the pelvis are symptoms of prostate cancer, but they are also, and most likely to be, symptoms of benign prostatic hyperplasia (BPH) or prostatitis.

In some men, the first symptoms of prostate cancer show up as severe pain in the back, a sign that the disease has spread to the bone and is life-threatening. Diagnosing prostate cancer for the first time when it is in its advanced stage is unusual today because of widespread screening for the disease.

Low free PSA and high bound PSA may indicate cancer

Before undergoing a biopsy based on PSA, ask your doctor how he is evaluating your PSA level.

The test you get when your blood is drawn is a total PSA, a combination of two forms called free PSA and bound PSA. Free PSA means it is not attached to a protein; bound means it is attached to a protein. Doctors can more clearly determine whether or not cancer is actually present by comparing the amount of free PSA to total PSA. Research shows that men with prostate cancer have a higher percentage of bound PSA and a lower percentage of free PSA in their blood. A low percentage of free PSA and a high percentage of bound PSA are indicative of cancer.

Research shows the ratio of free to total PSA helps distinguish between PSA elevations due to cancer and those caused by an enlarged prostate. Research indicates that using the percent of free PSA can help determine the need for biopsy and help decrease the amount of unnecessary biopsies being performed.

Studies indicate it is only necessary to perform a biopsy in men with total PSA levels between 4 and 10 when the percent of free PSA is 24 percent or lower. It would detect an estimated 90 percent of cancers and reduce unnecessary testing by 20 percent.

Is biopsy for you?

The typical sequence of events — and, if you're facing prostate cancer, the one that most likely got you to where you are today — begins when your annual physical shows your PSA has jumped from where it was last year and a digital rectal exam finds your prostate is slightly enlarged, so your family doctor refers you to a urologist.

The urologist performs the same exam, maybe even orders another PSA screening "just to make sure" and recommends a biopsy, which most men interpret as a "no choice" option.

You do, however, have the choice and it is in your best interest to inquire about your need for a biopsy so you don't end up undergoing an unnecessary painful and potentially risky procedure.

Doctors today pretty much agree that a biopsy should not be ordered solely on the reading of one number. A single number cannot define whether or not a man has prostate cancer because there really is no such thing as a "normal" PSA level. Most experts believe that PSA numbers should be used as part of an arsenal of information to determine if risk exists and if a biopsy should be undertaken. These variables include:

- results of a digital rectal examination. Have any nodules been detected?

- prostate size. Is it enlarged and has the man already been diagnosed with BPH?

- the difference in PSA at last test and at baseline, which is the level recorded at the first PSA.

- a man's age.

- hereditary factors. Have any relatives had cancer? What about race?

PSA and risk: what's your number?

The risk of discovering cancer on biopsy is:

PSA	Risk
0-2 ng/mL	12%
3-4 ng/mL	15-25%
5-10 ng/mL	17-32%
11-20 ng/mL	50-75%
21 ng/mL and higher	90%

Source: The Johns Hopkins White Papers: Prostate Disorders 2012

What to expect when you are expecting a biopsy

The time leading up to a biopsy can be a time of great anxiety for many men because they fear that a diagnosis of cancer is a foregone conclusion. Dr. Scholz and other proponents of a less aggressive approach to diagnosis and treatment believe this anxiety could be greatly reduced if men knew what to expect if the outcome is cancer. The majority of prostate cancers discovered today are low-risk disease, meaning they should be able to be safely monitored without treatment. Keep in mind about two-thirds of men over 60 have mostly low-grade prostate cancer even though it may be undiagnosed.

"Very few men understand what they are getting into when a biopsy is recommended," Dr. Scholz says in his book. "Family doctors and urologists schedule biopsies at the first sign of an elevated PSA, rarely educating their patients about what is likely to follow. Once a diagnosis of cancer is made, irrational fears drive most men into immediate radical therapy, even though low-risk prostate cancer is not life-threatening."

A biopsy involves inserting a small needle through the rectum and into the prostate to remove sample tissue for examination by a pathologist. The surgeon starts by doing a transrectal ultrasonography, called a TRUS, to determine the size of your prostate and identify areas that may be cancerous.

During the procedure you will be asked to lie on your side as an ultrasound probe about the size of a finger is gently inserted 3 to 4 inches into the rectum. The probe emits sound waves that are converted into video images corresponding with the different zones in the prostate. This gives the doctor a clear indication of your prostate's size.

Attached to the probe is a biopsy gun with a needle that is fired through the rectum wall and into the prostate where small pieces of tissue are extracted. The excisions all take place in less than a second.

Prostate cells don't grow like other cancers in one clump. Rather they form a particular pattern that can be readily spotted in the prostate's small environment. This is why doctors will take 10 or 12 tissue samples, what are called cores, which are sent to pathology for examination.

You will be given a local anesthesia, most likely lidocaine (Xylocaine), that should significantly lessen the pain and discomfort of the procedure. It also helps the doctor perform his job better because you won't be moving around too much.

The amount of pain you'll experience appears to be highly subjective. Some men complain of pain lasting up to a week after the procedures. Others don't complain at all. The extent of your discomfort depends a lot on your personal threshold for pain.

Can biopsy cause cancer?

The answer is a comforting and simple no.

At one time, biopsy carried the risk of spreading cancer if it was already present, but it is unheard of with the method used today.

Consider the results

It usually takes about a week before you get the results of your biopsy. Although biopsies are very good at scouting for cancer cells, they fail to spot cancer roughly 20 percent of the time, mostly in men with large prostates. When there is a suspicion of cancer and it doesn't show up in a biopsy, a doctor might order another one "just in case."

At times, biopsies reveal abnormal or atypical cells that might be suggestive of cancer but are not sufficient to make a definite diagnosis. In such cases, cancer is present in about 50 percent of the cases — another reason your doctor may suggest repeating the biopsy. Again, the choice is up to you.

"Unfortunately, doctors and patients alike still have the mistaken idea that time is of the essence," says Dr. Scholz. "This is true for other types of cancer, but it is rarely an issue with prostate cancer."

It's not cancer but ...

A biopsy that doesn't find cancer can detect premalignant lesions that can lead to cancer. Doctors call this high-grade prostatic intraepithelial neoplasia (HGPIN) and it can lead to finding cancer on a subsequent biopsy. A man with HGPIN has a 30 to 75 percent risk that these lesions will turn into cancer, depending on the number of lesions found on biopsy. Studies also show that lifestyle factors can influence this risk.

Biopsy is not risk-free

A biopsy can be risky business and in more ways than you might imagine. High on the need-to-know risk list is impotence. Two studies found that some men who had healthy sex lives before undergoing biopsy complained of impotence that lingered for months as a result of the procedure.

In one study, reported in the medical journal *Urology*, 41 percent of the men were not able to get an erection one month after the procedure and 15 percent of them still had the problem after six months. Another study, published in *The Journal of Urology*, reported 15 percent of men were unable to get an erection one month after having the test.

There are other risks, too. A new study found having a prostate biopsy more than doubled the risk of being hospitalized within the following month for infection, bleeding, or other complications.

Other research reports the rate of sepsis, a life-threatening bacterial infection of the blood, occurred in 3 percent of 2,023 men biopsied for prostate cancer. Sepsis is usually fatal if not promptly diagnosed and treated with hospitalization.

Three kinds of cancer

So the verdict is in and it's not the one you want to hear: You've got prostate cancer.

While a diagnosis of cancer is always devastating, prostate cancer offers a cushion of comfort not found with other common cancers, including lung, colon, and breast, because a great majority of prostate cancer is discovered in its early stage.

More and more of the best doctors today see prostate cancer as three states and base their treatment recommendation on risk. The three states of prostate cancer based on risk are:

- low-risk, or early-stage cancer, which can generally be monitored through active surveillance

- intermediate-risk cancer, which is considered a higher risk but can be treated with less aggressive treatments that can include active surveillance

- high-risk cancer, which calls for some kind of aggressive treatment

Cancer grade is based on six variables and the findings within those variables. Of course, there may be overlap of some of the variable metrics within these broad types.

Cancer type	Gleason score	% biopsy cores with cancer	PSA level	PSA density	PSA velocity	Digital rectal exam
Low-risk	Less than 7	Less than 34%	Less than 10	Less than 0.15	Less than 2	No nodule
Intermediate-risk	7	35-50%	11-20	More than 0.15	Less than 2	Small nodule
High-risk	8 and higher	More than 50%	21 and higher	More than 0.15	More than 2	Larger nodule

Gleason score

Your score on the Gleason Grading System is considered one of the most important factors in deciding your cancer type. It is based on tumor grade, determined in pathology examination, which indicates to what extent the structure of the tumor cells found in the biopsy deviate from normal. The system is named after Dr. Donald F. Gleason, who devised it in 1966.

Normal cells are highly organized structures with clearly defined borders and clear centers. By contrast, cancer cells display various degrees of distortion and differentiation. Those that are closest to normal are classified as Grade 1 and those that are the most irregular and disorganized are classified as Grade 5.

The Gleason score is determined by identifying and giving a classification to the two most prevalent organizational patterns found in the tumor cells and adding the two together. For example, if the most common pattern is a Grade 2 and the second most common pattern is a Grade 4, your Gleason score would be a 6. Gleason scores range from 2 through 10. At one time, all Gleason scores were targeted for some type of treatment, however today, scores 2 through 5 are not considered to be distinctive enough to be of concern.

Percent of biopsy cores with cancer

During a biopsy, approximately a dozen tissue samples are taken. The percent of those that are cancerous are weighted toward your risk.

PSA level

Prostate-specific antigen, better known as PSA, measures an enzyme produced almost exclusively by the glandular cells of the prostate. Normally, only very small amounts are present in the blood. High levels of PSA in the blood indicate that there is something abnormal occurring in the prostate and these abnormalities include prostate cancer.

PSA density

One of the reasons the PSA test can give incorrect results is because prostate glands come in all sizes. A broad rule is that larger prostates produce more PSA than smaller ones. Therefore, a high PSA reading could simply mean you have a large, but normal, prostate. To fix this problem, doctors measure the size or volume of your prostate with a transrectal ultrasound and divide the PSA by this number. The result is your PSA density, or the amount of PSA produced per gram of prostate. The higher your PSA density, the greater your risk of cancer. Research suggests that a PSA density greater than 0.15 indicates a high risk of cancer.

PSA velocity

PSA velocity takes into account annual changes in PSA levels. PSA levels rise slowly in men with BPH and more rapidly in men with cancer. PSA elevation from BPH usually occurs at the rate of less than one-half point a year. Men with low-risk cancer also have slowly rising PSA levels. Aggressive cancer grows more rapidly, resulting in larger annual changes in PSA velocity. Studies indicate a rise of two points in one year is a strong indication that aggressive cancer might be present.

A study at Johns Hopkins University School of Medicine found that a PSA increase of more than 0.75 per year was an early predictor of prostate cancer in men with PSA levels between 4 and 10.

PSA velocity is helpful in detecting early cancer in men with mildly elevated PSA levels when a digital rectal exam does not find anything abnormal.

Digital rectal examination

This test, which is typically part of a man's annual physical, is a manual exam in which the doctor inserts a lubricated gloved finger about an inch to an inch and a half into the rectum to feel the prostate to detect if the gland is enlarged or has suspicious hardness.

How tumor grade is determined

How advanced a cancer appears to be is based on the grade of the tumor. There is a clinical grade and a pathological grade.

Clinical grade is based on your doctor's educated opinion as a result of what he finds when he performs a digital rectal exam and gets the results of your PSA test and biopsy. The three tests give him a pretty good idea of what kind of a tumor he's dealing with.

The "official" or pathological grade of the tumor cannot be determined until a pathologist exams the tumor itself after surgery. There is also another way to get a pathological grading on a tumor before or without surgery by using a mathematical formula called Partin Tables.

Partin Tables, named after Johns Hopkins urologist Alan W. Partin, M.D., Ph.D., who helped develop them, are based on data collected from nearly 6,000 men who were treated for prostate cancer at Johns Hopkins from 2000 to 2005.

Keep in mind that there is a difference between clinical and pathological findings should you hear words such as "clinical grade" or "Partin Tables" being thrown around when your doctor is talking to you or with other medical experts about your tumor. If you're looking at a written chart, you might also see a lowercase "p" or "c" in front of the grade. A "c" before a tumor grade — for example, cT1 — indicates clinical grade. A "p" before the tumor grade means pathological grade, the one that counts the most.

Tumor grading is based on a system called TNM, which stands for tumor, nodes, and metastases. These are the classifications and what they mean.

TNM cancer grading system

Tumor Grade	Description
T1	Tumor cannot be felt on digital rectal exam (DRE) or seen with diagnostic imaging.
T1a	Tumor found incidentally during surgery for BPH and is present in less than 5% of removed tissues.
T1b	Tumor found incidentally during surgery for BPH and involves more than 5% of removed tissue.
T1c	Tumor found during biopsy performed because of elevated PSA.
T2	Tumor can be felt during DRE but is believed to be confined to the gland.
T2a	Tumor confined to one-half or less of one side of the prostate.
T2b	Tumor involves more than one-half of one side of the prostate.
T2c	Tumor involves both sides of the prostate.

TNM cancer grading system *continued*

Tumor Grade	Description
T3	Tumor extends through the prostate capsule and may involve the seminal vesicles.
T3a	Tumor extends through the prostate capsule but does not involve the seminal vesicles.
T3b	Tumor has spread to the seminal vesicles.
T4	Tumor has invaded adjacent structures other than the seminal vesicles — bladder neck, pelvic wall, or rectum.
N0	Cancer has not spread to lymph nodes.
N1	Tumor has spread to lymph nodes in the pelvic region.
M0	Cancer has not spread to other organs.
M1	Cancer has spread to distant organs.
M1a	Cancer has spread to distant lymph nodes.
M1b	Cancer has spread to the bones.
M1c	Cancer has spread to other organs, which may or may not include the bones.

Source: National Cancer Institute

Tests and more tests

Depending on what your doctor determines about your tumor, or perhaps just for assurance, he may order a few more tests. These are among them.

Bone scan

Technically known as a radionuclide scintigraphy, a bone scan is the most sensitive way to spot changes within the bones.

With this test you will be injected with a harmless radioactive substance and asked to lie on a table while a special camera takes pictures of your bone structure. The test can take up to 45 minutes. Afterward, a radiologist will read the films looking for hot spots that could possibly indicate cancer.

The test can only identify biological changes in bone and cannot ascertain the cause. Other than cancer, osteoporosis and other diseases could show up as hot spots.

Some physicians will not bother with a bone scan for men with a PSA less than 10 because the possibility that it has spread to the bone is unlikely. Other doctors will order the test so the likelihood can be ruled out.

PCA-3 urine test

This is a relatively new test that measures ribonucleic acid (RNA) secreted by cancer cells into the urine following manual massage of the prostate. The amount of suspicious RNA in the urine increases in proportion to both the size and aggressiveness of a man's cancer. Unlike PSA, PCA-3 is not affected by prostate size. Low amounts of PCA-3 in the urine, say less than 40, send a strong signal that specific amounts of aggressive cells are unlikely.

PCA-3, like blood pressure readings, can vary from test to test. When doctors use this test, they generally use the average of several tests taken over the course of six months.

Spectrographic endorectal magnetic resonance imaging

This is a state-of-the-art MRI in which a coil within an inflated latex balloon is positioned in the rectum to generate clear and detailed three-dimensional pictures of the prostate. It also provides important metabolic information about prostate cancer. For example, it can detect the ratio of substances called citrate and choline in cells. A high level of choline and a low citrate level indicate the presence of cancer. This test also provides a more precise measurement of prostate size.

Prior to taking the test, you must fast for 24 hours and cleanse the system with an enema. You will be offered a sedative, as confinement in an MRI machine makes many people claustrophobic.

Ask the crucial questions

The possibility of having cancer is nerve-wracking, but you'll be in a much better frame of mind to ask important questions about the outcome of a biopsy before it is performed.

Accurate information about cancer is essential for deciding how to treat the cancer. Ask plenty of questions. How big is the tumor? Does the cancer penetrate the capsule wall? Even more important, is the cancer growing?

Make sure you have all the critical numbers discussed in this chapter before you begin discussing your treatment options. If they aren't offered to you, request them. Your doctor is obligated to give you access to your records and should be willing to share them and discuss them with you.

Once you have all your essential information, you'll be in a much better position to reach the best decision concerning your treatment options. The options available for managing prostate cancer, along with their pros and cons, are discussed in the next chapter.

Prostate cancer: the wise man's guide to making the right decision

Every man is different — his lifestyle, his mindset, his health, and even his prostate. They all need to be taken into account when considering a treatment for prostate cancer.

A diagnosis of cancer is frightening and can instill you with unrelenting anxiety. This is understandable. Go into any support group and you'll hear stories about men who have been railroaded into unnecessary, aggressive treatment because a doctor or other well-meaning person scared them half to death with the idea that forgoing surgery was putting one foot in the grave.

It's unfathomable to hear the diagnosis of cancer and not think about treating it. Yet, it is exactly what you should be thinking about because you could be among the estimated 56 percent of men each year who are diagnosed with prostate cancer that is so insignificant it most likely will never be a threat during their lifetime — what doctors now recognize as low-risk, or favorable-risk, cancer.

"Most men with favorable-risk prostate cancer are not destined to die of their disease, even in the absence of treatment," says Laurence

Klotz, M.D., chief of urology at Sunnybrook Health Science Center in Toronto and one of the leading critics of overdiagnosis and overtreatment of the disease.

Most people — and this includes many doctors — are of a mind that every type of cancer is so ominous that it must be caught early and treated aggressively to avoid what would otherwise be a painful and premature death. "This widely shared preconception often leads the patient to make a quick and early decision for treatment, regardless of the risks and benefits," says Dr. Klotz. "For some cancers this fear is warranted, but for most men with favorable-risk prostate cancer, their condition is far removed from that of a rampaging, aggressive disease."

By no means is this meant to dissuade you from having surgery if you and your doctor decide you need it, but keep in mind that over-diagnosis and overtreatment of prostate cancer is a proven reality.

Aggressive treatment, including prostate surgery, is driven by profit and by the unpleasant legal environment that means doctors can be sued for not quickly treating a condition that later proves to be fatal.

Remember, the majority of men who are diagnosed with prostate cancer have nonthreatening, low-risk disease, yet 90 percent of them are given aggressive treatments that carry a high risk of life-altering consequences. All men who have their prostate surgically removed will experience impotence and incontinence at least temporarily and it's anyone's guess who will permanently end up with one or the other — or both. Once the prostate is removed, there is no going back. It is impossible to undo harm that has been done.

Current trend: less aggressive treatment

"An argument can be made that the overdiagnosis of prostate cancer is problematic primarily to the extent that it leads to overtreatment," the American Cancer Society (ACS) said in a review article published in the journal *Cancer* that cautions doctors to proceed cautiously when recommending treatment.

In the most simplistic terms, experts say, only men with aggressive cancer should get aggressive treatment and doctors should fully inform men with low-risk disease of the most benign option — active surveillance, meaning no treatment at all. Men "in the middle" — those with intermediate-stage disease — have the toughest decision. They are the ones stuck with the nagging questions that are often difficult to answer: *Is aggressive treatment really necessary? What am I risking if I just wait a little longer? Is it possible that my cancer is growing so slowly that I could safely delay treatment for years?*

The challenge for doctors, says the ACS, is to be able to differentiate between prostate cancer that should be treated and cancer that should be left alone. Your challenge is to make sure you get all the need-to-know information about your disease and an honest, candid, and unbiased account of all treatment options from your doctor.

Remember, prostate cancer is slow-growing. Unless you're among the rare few with aggressive cancer caught in a late stage, time is on your side. For your own protection, your first decision is to make no decision until you are able to make an informed, rational, and unemotional one. So take a deep breath, ease your emotions, and let knowledge and common sense be your guide.

How slow can prostate cancer grow?

Doctors first started to realize the slow motion of prostate cancer progression when autopsies of men dying from causes other than cancer found tumors in the prostates of young men with no history of prostate problems. They found cancer in 30 percent of men in their 30s and in more than 50 percent of men over age 50. This led to the discovery that prostate cancer starts to grow in men during their 20s and 30s and can remain harmless for decades.

"That observation is startling in the context of the typical age of death from prostate cancer — about 80 years," says Dr. Klotz. "It implies a 50-year time course from inception to mortality!"

For most patients with prostate cancer that eventually becomes life-threatening, explains Dr. Klotz, this means a period of slow undetected tumor progression that takes at least 20 years, followed by another period of slow progression spanning 15 years or more from diagnosis to metastasis to death.

"The implication is that most patients have a long window of curability," he says. This is especially true for men with low-risk disease. "It also implies that young age at diagnosis should not preclude a surveillance approach."

This, however, is not the way doctors have been trained to view active surveillance. Traditionally, this approach has been considered an option best reserved for older men, who would die of something else before prostate cancer had a chance to get them. An emerging trend is reversing this mindset, although it, too, is slow-growing.

Is your doctor being straight with you?

Prostate cancer is different from other cancers in many ways, including who treats it. Early-stage disease is almost always diagnosed by a urologist who is a surgeon. This is what the urologist likely does for a living. It's the main reason why surgery is the most frequently used treatment option, even for low-risk cases.

Cancer specialists, called oncologists, may recommend a variety of treatments for cancer but are rarely involved in treating early prostate cancer. The subspecialty of prostate oncology is quite rare. Out of the approximately 10,000 oncologists in the United States, only around 100 of them specialize in prostate cancer.

In the next chapter, you'll learn how to work with your urologist to assure you get the best treatment.

Active surveillance: watch and wait

Active surveillance is exactly what it sounds like — doing nothing except seeing your doctor on a regular schedule and getting periodic tests to find out if your prostate cancer is advancing. Treatment is only considered if and when the cancer becomes a risk. And, since there are no treatments yet available without quality-of-life issues, waiting means a better treatment could surface by the time you actually need it. Or, it's possible you may go the rest of your life without needing aggressive treatment.

This is *not* like playing Russian roulette with cancer. Even the ACS cautions doctors to be open-minded about offering it as an option — and for good reason. Credible statistics recently released reveal that an estimated *90 percent* of men who safely qualify for active surveillance end up getting radical surgery instead.

A startling statistic, for sure, which leads to the question: Why? It is not because doctors are practicing bad medicine or doing it for the money. Dr. Klotz, among other experts, believes that, when it comes to cancer, doctors, and especially surgeons, have an inherent resistance to the idea of not treating it. After all, their medical training is all about *treating* disease, not watching it. They instinctively feel safe within the established protocols of traditional medicine. Then there is the other ugly fact they rightfully fear — a malpractice lawsuit.

"The reasons behind what is likely underutilization of active surveillance are multiple and complex," concedes the ACS in the *Cancer* article, adding that it is not just doctors, but also patients who are reticent about delaying treatment, though for a different reason — reflexive fear. The medical literature, however, cites scores of studies that show the fear associated with a wait-and-see approach is unfounded. The preponderance of evidence shows that active

> Imagine you have a disease that might eventually require amputation of a leg in a small percentage of those who have that disease. Would you be better off if you had that leg amputated as soon as possible if there was no increased risk in waiting?

surveillance, when conducted properly and selected by the right candidates, poses no greater risk of early death from cancer than it does to men who have surgery immediately.

Even at Johns Hopkins, where possibly more radical prostatectomies are performed a year than at any other institution, doctors agree there is no need for men with low risk to rush to surgery. "Our data suggest that patients with low-risk cancer can be reassured that immediate treatment is not necessary," Hopkins researchers reported in *The Journal of Urology*.

Is active surveillance for you?

Even with the assurance of the world's best doctors, there are no absolutes when it comes to forgoing treatment in favor of having no treatment. However, the ACS, assisted by the country's top prostate cancer experts, has come up with a profile of the ideal candidate. It is a man with:

- a Gleason score of 6 or less, with no single tumor pattern that measures 4 or 5.

- a PSA under 10.

- tumor density on biopsy cores totaling less than 33 percent.

- no single biopsy core greater than 50 percent.

- tumor stage that does not exceed T1 to T2a.

At one time, active surveillance was only considered a wise option for older men meeting these parameters, but this is no longer the case. Men of all ages are candidates to have many more years without disability if they meet the criteria.

Guidelines for active surveillance

If you choose active surveillance you will be expected to see your doctor routinely and have certain tests, which at times may mean more biopsies. You and your doctor should re-evaluate this approach if your cancer ever progresses to a stage where treatment is the better option.

The recommended timelines for watching your cancer differ slightly from one treatment center to another, but they all involve the same surveillance techniques. The ACS and many top treatment hospitals recommend this protocol for active surveillance:

- a repeat PSA and digital rectal exam every six months

- a confirming biopsy within the first year of diagnosis and repeat biopsies every three to five years until age 80

- optional spectrographic endorectal MRI

Some doctors and institutions also recommend:

- a baseline color Doppler ultrasound, which is repeated every six months.

- a baseline PSA-3 urine sample, which is repeated every six to 12 months.

- an annual spectrographic endorectal ultrasound.

With active surveillance, experts agree, men still have plenty of opportunity to get treatment without putting their lives at risk. When you are working closely with a doctor who supports active surveillance, treatment can be started at the first sign of cancer progression while the disease is still curable.

The time to start considering treatment is if and when:

- PSA doubles in less than three years. This occurs in about 20 percent of men who opt for active surveillance.

- a repeat biopsy shows that the cancer has progressed to a Gleason score of 7, especially if one tumor pattern measures a 4 on the 5-point scale. This occurs in approximately 5 percent of men who opt for active surveillance.

Also, men on active surveillance should contact their doctors if they experience any of these symptoms that may indicate the cancer has become aggressive:

- blood in the urine

- difficulty urinating

- pain in the pelvic area or lower back

The emotional side of waiting

What does having prostate cancer and doing nothing about it do to the psyche? About the same thing it does to men diagnosed with prostate cancer who have surgery, studies show. It raises your anxiety. Men who don't have any treatment worry about cancer progressing just as much as men who've had surgery worry about the cancer coming back.

"Surveillance may be stressful for some men, but the reality is that most patients with prostate cancer, whether treated or not, are concerned about the risk of progression," says Laurence Klotz, M.D.

Bottom line: Don't let worry and fear dissuade you from opting for active surveillance if you are a candidate for nontreatment. You are likely to be just as anxious about the cancer coming back after surgery. And you'll be a lot better off treating the anxiety with stress-reduction techniques than thinking that having surgery will relieve the anxiety.

Time and safety are on your side

What's the risk of waiting? For most men, there is none, according to ongoing studies that have been following thousands of men who have been on active surveillance for at least 10 years.

"Prostate cancer mortality is exceptionally low," Dr. Klotz reported in the journal *Current Oncology* after reviewing the results of these studies. In most men on active surveillance, death eventually results from other causes unrelated to prostate cancer.

Other studies report no added risk for men who delayed treatment for more than two years. These studies "suggest that well-characterized, early-stage tumors followed by experienced physicians and knowledgeable patients do not progress rapidly and deferring treatment appears not to alter their natural history," says the ACS.

One study conducted by Johns Hopkins' Ballentine Carter, M.D., who is considered one of the world's leading prostate cancer experts, specifically evaluated men under active surveillance whose cancer eventually progressed to the point where radical surgery was advised. He found the men who delayed treatment were no worse off than the men who had immediate treatment.

Other studies have found similar results. One study conducted at Sloan-Kettering Cancer Center in New York City found that half of the men who selected active surveillance had no further progression of their cancer after 10 years. Of those whose cancer advanced and were then treated, the cancer came back in only one man during the 10 years. "Men with low-grade prostate cancer can elect active surveillance and have excellent long-term results," reported the researchers.

Surgery: out with the prostate

You've heard of it as a radical prostatectomy, nerve-sparing prostatectomy, laparoscopic prostatectomy, and robotic prostatectomy, but they all boil down to the same thing: surgical removal of the prostate. Though one surgery attempts to spare your sex life and another claims to minimize side effects, the differences among them are more like splitting hairs. Scientific scrutiny has found there is no procedure that will leave you unscathed.

No matter which surgical method you choose, the best advice for the best outcome, studies show, is to find a highly skilled surgeon.

Choose someone who has done the procedure a lot and with great success. The prostate is located in tight quarters in the pelvic region, within millimeters of the bladder and rectum, so there virtually is no room for a slip of the scalpel. Also, a lot of blood surges through the prostate, so there is generally a lot of blood involved in the surgery, which can create a visual challenge, especially with nerve-sparing surgery, the type aimed at preserving your long-term sex life.

If at all possible, find a medical center devoted to cancer treatment and prostate cancer in particular. This is where you'll find state-of-the-art diagnostic techniques and practitioners who specialize in specific prostate cancer procedures. You'll find a list of the top centers on page 342.

While surgery is billed as a cure for prostate cancer, it is only a cure if all the cancer is removed. Even the world's best surgeons leave undetected cancer behind some of the time. After surgery is when PSA plays a crucial role — the role, by the way, for which it was originally intended. It can detect if the cancer is coming back.

The surgical trifecta

The best possible outcome after radical prostatectomy is what researchers at Memorial Sloan-Kettering Cancer Center in New York City call a surgical trifecta: Freedom from recurrence of cancer, complete recovery of continence, and complete restoration of erections.

So what are the odds of winning the trifecta when you're gambling your quality of life on a radical prostatectomy to beat prostate cancer? After observing the surgical outcomes of more than 1,500 men who underwent the procedure at Sloan-Kettering over the course of six years, researchers called it at 62 percent.

Keep in mind these results are from one of the very best cancer centers. Most outcomes may not be this good.

Seldom-spoken risks

Impotence and incontinence understandably are the greatest concerns for men undergoing a prostatectomy. Science has yet to design a surgical procedure where these concerns are nonexistent. As difficult as impotence and incontinence are to accept, there are other lesser-known risks that should concern you as well. The unfortunate truth is that complications from prostate cancer surgery are even higher than previously thought, according to studies reported in the journal *Urology* and the *Journal of the American Medical Association* (*JAMA*).

The *Urology* study, which followed 101,604 men who had undergone a radical prostatectomy, found the rate of serious problems after surgery averaged 24 percent and went up with a man's age. "Complications and readmission after prostatectomy are substantially more common than previously recognized," the study concluded.

Exactly what did these studies find? The need for blood transfusions due to blood loss during surgery was as high as 20 percent. The complication rate one month after surgery was 20 percent and half of the problems involved the heart, lungs, and blood vessels. After three months, readmission to the hospital due to complications of radical prostatectomy was about 9 percent. Many of these complications can be fatal. Generally, the risk of dying during or soon after surgery is understated.

Here is what else you need to know about the risks associated with radical prostatectomy.

Higher rates of impotence. Impotence rates of 50 percent by even the best surgeons are reported. Even men who fully recover their ability to have an erection after nerve-sparing surgery undergo a protracted period of impotence often lasting up to one or two years. Longer-term impotence after nerve-sparing surgery is about 27 percent, according to the *JAMA* study.

Incredible shrinking penis. The side effect most likely not to get discussed before surgery? Expect your penis to shrink. It's kind of like the use-it-or-lose-it theory. A muscle that isn't used, or in the after-surgery scenario, one that doesn't want to work, atrophies and gets smaller.

The proof was found in 124 Florida men who agreed to have their penises measured while flaccid before and after undergoing a radical prostatectomy. The penises in all the men were "significantly smaller after surgery" and nerve-sparing surgery made no difference, reported the researchers in *The Journal of Urology*. The average shrinkage was a half inch, but it was "much greater" in many of the men.

Medically assisted erections. Men can be led to believe, or simply choose to believe, that successful surgery that spares the nerves means their love life will simply resume as normal. Unfortunately, this is not the way it works. Not only does it take time — often a year or longer — to regain the ability to have an erection, but it most likely means help from expensive prescription drugs or medical devices.

Time in diapers. All men who undergo surgery leave the hospital with a catheter inserted through the penis into the bladder. The urethra, which runs through the prostate, takes a beating during surgery. The prostate comes out, but the urethra stays, so it must be separated from the prostate and reconnected to the bladder. This requires healing time in which the urethra doesn't do you a bit of good. Hence, the catheter. Even after the catheter is removed, the urethra requires some retraining, so expect to spend time wearing adult diapers for anywhere from a few weeks to a few months. An estimated 12 to 16 percent of men have some degree of permanent urinary leakage, according to *JAMA*, and about 10 percent of them will have urinary symptoms severe enough to require more surgery.

Hard-as-a-rock urethra. Another complication is the formation of scar tissue around the urethra at the site where it is reconnected to the bladder. The condition is called urinary stricture, and it makes urination very painful. It can also make urination impossible, a medical emergency called urinary retention.

Urinary stricture can be corrected in a procedure called urethral dilation, in which probes are inserted through the penis to expand the rock-hard tissue near the bladder. Although the procedure allows you to release urine without pain or difficulty, it virtually guarantees you'll be left incontinent.

Going to extremes: a tale of two treatments

There hasn't been a lot of scientific scrutiny comparing the outcome of surgery versus no treatment because it's not all that easy to find a large group of men with cancer who are willing to put their destiny on the line based, essentially, on the flip of a coin. However, in 1989 Swedish researchers managed to recruit 695 men with early-stage cancer who agreed to such an experiment. The men were randomly assigned to either have a radical prostatectomy or have no immediate treatment at all.

Twelve years later, 12.5 percent of the men who had their prostate removed died of prostate cancer compared to 18 percent of the men who underwent watchful waiting. Although the death rate in the men who had surgery was lower, the researchers said the almost 6 percent difference was not "statistically significant" — meaning it was virtually a tie. The only difference is the surgery itself put the men at higher risk of complications, including death.

Leaving cancer behind. Even the best doctors can leave cancer behind, according to a study in *The Journal of Urology*. The study examined the outcomes of surgery at two prestigious medical centers in New York City and Seattle, and found the top-rated doctors left cancer behind in 10 percent of operations. The rate ranged from 11 percent to 48 percent among other doctors.

Leaving cancer behind is not usually a sign of physician error. Standard radiology imaging techniques used today cannot detect microscopic residual disease. This is why doctors cut beyond the perimeter of cancer to help ensure that any undetected residual cancer is extracted.

Now that you know the risks of surgery, here are the essential differences among the techniques available today.

Radical prostatectomy: popular by 'demand'

Radical prostatectomy, also known as open prostatectomy, has been considered the ultimate cure for prostate cancer for 100 years. Today, it is considered radical in more ways than one. Most notoriously, it is the most widely used treatment option no matter how serious or benign the disease. New research reveals that 90 percent of men with prostate cancer that probably never would have advanced enough to become life-threatening even without treatment end up getting this life-altering surgery. It is not something you want to agree to without careful consideration and deliberation.

Urologists argue for it, because it is considered a cure for the disease. Cynical opponents of the surgery say urologists argue for it because urologists are surgeons! Nevertheless, it is only a cure if all the cancer is caught. Even when the prostate is removed, it is not a given that undetected cancer will not be left behind.

A surgeon removes the prostate in one of two approaches. The most common approach, called retropubic radical prostatectomy, involves getting to the prostate by making a cut in the lower abdomen from the pubic bone to the navel. In a perineal radical prostatectomy, the surgeon reaches the prostate through the perineum, the area between the scrotum and rectum. This technique is usually reserved for older men or men in poor health who have a higher risk of complications.

Before the prostate is removed, the surgeon will do a biopsy of the lymph nodes closest to the prostate to find out if there is evidence the cancer has spread. Depending on the doctor, this can be done through a minimally invasive procedure using a fine instrument called a laparoscope prior to surgery, or it can be done at the beginning of the surgery before the prostate is removed. If cancer is found in the lymph nodes, the surgeon most likely will cancel the operation because there's no use in removing the prostate if cancer has already spread.

If the pathologist gives the surgeon the green light, the surgeon will begin to remove the prostate by cutting it loose from the surrounding tissue. The seminal vesicles and vas deferens, the main ducts that carry semen to its destination, will also be taken out. This means that you'll be unable to produce semen again.

To minimize bleeding, which can obscure the line of vision, the surgeon cuts and ties off the group of veins that lie at the top of the prostate and urethra. The surgeon then severs the urethra from the prostate, taking care to avoid cutting the sphincter muscle that controls your ability to start and stop urine flow.

The last step is to detach the prostate from the bladder and urethra. The surgeon cuts a hole in the bottom of the bladder about the size of a quarter. He uses sutures to close the opening to about the size of a dime, then pulls the urethra into position and stitches the two together.

Once you're healed, urine will run from the bladder straight into the urethra instead of going through the prostatic urethra that was once part of the prostate. In order for the new connection between the urethra and bladder to heal, a catheter is inserted through the penis and into the bladder to collect urine. You'll leave the hospital with the device in place, where it will remain for two or three weeks. You can expect to be temporarily incontinent when the device is removed.

The procedure takes anywhere from 90 minutes to three hours depending on the skill of the surgeon and the size of the prostate. It requires general anesthesia and you'll be in the hospital anywhere from four days to a week. Full recovery can take three months.

A small percentage of patients will die during or soon after surgery. Death rates are related to the skill of the surgeon and the reputation of the hospital.

Although most men eventually regain urinary control, it's impossible to predict how long it will take. It can vary from a few weeks to up to a year. Studies show that about 50 percent of men regain urinary control in about three months. You can read about the complications of incontinence and how to control it in Chapter 7.

A different kind of orgasm

Removing the prostate is the male version of a female hysterectomy. It means no babies. It also means a different kind of orgasm.

When the prostate is removed, the surgeon also takes out the seminal vesicles, ducts involved in mixing sperm with other fluid to fertilize the female egg when you ejaculate. Without the seminal vesicles and prostate, there is no ejaculatory fluid. You can have an orgasm, but it is called a dry orgasm. Lack of a prostate does not stifle sexual interest. Good news: you can have an orgasm without having an erection.

Nerve-sparing prostatectomy: the big gamble

Until the early 1980s, when doctors removed the prostate everything went with it, including your ability to ever have an erection again. The person who changed all that and made erections possible without a prostate is Patrick Walsh, M.D., urologist-in-chief at Johns Hopkins University Medical Center. He developed a technique to spare the neurovascular bundles, two sets of nerves located on each side of the prostate that are responsible for activating the penis into position. A strong erection is necessary for vaginal penetration. Sparing even one set of nerves makes having an erection possible.

Dr. Walsh's nerve-sparing technique made him world-famous and the hero of men with prostate cancer. It's an incredible feat, especially when you consider erection-making nerves are the size of a strand of hair, making them invisible to the naked eye. Complicating the ability to leave them intact is the amount of blood involved in taking out the prostate. So you can understand why saving the nerves cannot be a full-fledged promise, even from the best of doctors.

But sacrificing the nerves during nerve-sparing surgery is less likely to be caused by a slip of the scalpel than it is by the location of the cancer. Surgeons need to cut outside the margins of the cancer to ensure that they get it all, meaning if the cancer is involved anywhere near the nerves, out they go. You may go under anesthesia counting the days until your next erection, but wake up to find out your chances of it happening are zero.

In nerve-sparing surgery, the physician follows the same procedure as with a radical prostatectomy. Once the urethra is separated from the prostate and bladder, the surgeon carefully dissects the nerves away from the prostate before cutting through the bladder neck to sever the prostate.

The nerve-sparing technique is also easier on the urethra and studies show there is a lower risk of urinary complications and incontinence as a result of the surgery.

Every sexually active man undergoing a radical prostatectomy desires surgery to spare the nerves. Nevertheless, no matter what you're told or how expert your surgeon is, whether or not you'll eventually emerge as your former sexual self is hard to predict. At best, the odds that you'll eventually recover complete erectile function have been reported to be anywhere from 16 to 76 percent, though some doctors claim a success rate closer to 90 percent or even more. Also, keep in mind that recovery doesn't happen overnight. Nor is it spontaneous. Many men find it is a struggle and requires the support of drugs like sildenafil (Viagra).

Unfortunately, the older you are, the less likely it is that this procedure will be effective. An estimated 70 to 90 percent of men age 50 and younger eventually end up regaining their potency after successful nerve-sparing surgery. For men ages 60 to 70, the percentage is around 58 percent — and some experts warn that this is being optimistic. According to reports issued by Johns Hopkins, where the procedure was designed, the risk of impotence depends a lot on a man's age, the quality of erections prior to surgery, and the surgeon's skill.

"The majority of men who have good-quality erections before surgery and a skillfully performed operation have return of erectile functions," said Dr. Carter in *The Johns Hopkins White Papers Prostate Disorders 2010.* "Full recovery can take more than a year in some instances, however." Men who have trouble having erections as a result of surgery may be able to find success with drugs for erectile dysfunction.

When a shot of radiation helps

A course of radiation after surgery appears to help extend longevity and reduce the risk of cancer spreading in men with locally advanced cancer, meaning the cancer extends throughout the gland and may even possibly have invaded the seminal vesicles, according to the results of a long-term study.

For the study, researchers divided men with advanced localized cancer who had undergone a radical prostatectomy into two groups. One group underwent radiation therapy shortly after the surgery. Men in the other group received radiation only when there was evidence that the cancer was coming back. After 13 years, men who received radiation after surgery were 29 percent less likely to have cancer recur and spread and 28 percent less likely to die from the disease than men who waited until the cancer returned to get the radiation.

Laparoscopic radical prostatectomy: the 'minimalist'

Laparoscopes have changed the landscape of surgery, making it less invasive and offering the patient a faster recovery. Some doctors and medical centers offer it as an option to open radical surgery. As surgery goes, the option is alluring. Rather than making a large incision, the surgeon makes tiny cuts in the abdomen near the belly button and uses a camera-guided fine instrument to make the maneuvers required to remove the prostate. The scope offers the surgeon a magnified visual image 10 to 15 times greater than what can be seen with the naked eye, a great advantage when the goal is sparing the nerves.

The primary advantage of it all is in favor of the patient: less pain and blood loss, minimal scarring, a lower risk of infection, less time with a catheter, and a faster recovery time. The average hospital stay is two days compared to a week with open surgery and recovery time is one to two weeks compared to three months.

So far, so good, you could say. After all, who wouldn't opt for less risk and a speedier recovery when all else is considered equal! There is, however, a big unknown — the lack of studies showing whether the laparoscope works better than standard surgery at what really matters most — getting all the cancer so there is no recurrence of the disease five or 10 years down the road. Also, at best, laparoscopic surgery carries the same sexual and urinary side effects as open surgery, though some studies indicate the risk is actually higher.

The biggest criticism of the procedure is the lack of the physician's physical contact with the prostate. A great deal of a surgeon's skill is his literal feel for the gland. Surgeons use their fingers to feel the prostate during traditional surgery to define how much they must cut to capture all the cancer and achieve the best possible outcome. Cancer cells produce changes in tissue firmness that surgeons can sense as they feel what they cannot always see — what they call tactile feedback.

This means urologists have to acquire a new set of skills to perform the laparoscopic operation and go through the learning curve that goes with it. There is a financial incentive to do so, because laser surgery is more expensive and doctors can bill a higher cost to insurance companies. The incentive for the insurance companies is that the surgery reduces the risk of the complications that can develop during and after surgery and the costs that would go with it. It's a win-win situation for all — almost.

There are downsides to a laparoscopic prostatectomy in addition to the lack of long-term studies on its safety. For one, the surgery takes more time than open surgery, usually around three to four hours or even more, depending on the

> Men undergoing a laparoscopic prostatectomy had a threefold greater risk of needing additional treatment later on than men who underwent traditional surgery.

surgeon's skill and the complexity of the cancer. This also means you'd have to spend more time under anesthesia, which carries a risk of its own. Another risk is that the surgeon might need to revert to standard surgery if difficulty is encountered during the procedure. One study, reported in the *Journal of Clinical Oncology*, found men had a threefold greater risk of needing additional treatment later on than men who underwent traditional surgery.

Another consideration is that the surgery appears to be going out of style, as it is being overshadowed by a more advanced procedure that made its debut in the United States in 2000 — laparoscopic prostatectomy performed by a robot.

Robotic prostatectomy: hands-off surgery

If you're timid about trusting your prostate to man, will you have more faith in a robot? Apparently many men do because the demand for robotic prostatectomy is sky-high. According to a 2010 article in *The Wall Street Journal*, medical centers that do not offer the surgery are losing business to hospitals that do. Statistics show that more than 85 percent of prostates are taken out these days by means of robotic-assisted surgery, mostly due to patient demand.

The focus of all the fanfare is the revolutionary Da Vinci Surgical System. With the system, your surgeon doesn't get anywhere near your prostate. He may not even be in the same room! However, the surgeon does control the robot doing the job, so the robot really is only as good as the surgeon manipulating the robotic arms. A great deal of skill is required to learn the procedure. And lots of practice is needed to become proficient.

In robotic surgery, the surgeon sits behind a console and looks through a set of three-dimensional, high-definition goggles while maneuvering mechanical arms with tips the size of a dime that do what a surgeon would otherwise do with his hands — but better. In addition to superior three-dimensional vision, the robot offers enhanced dexterity that allows surgical instruments to rotate in ways not possible with human hands and fingers in such a small space. The manufacturer of the Da Vinci System says it offers intuitive precision and control with state-of-the-art surgical dissecting and suturing capabilities.

More hype than performance?

The big draw of robotic surgery has a lot more to do with good marketing than it does with being the latest and greatest way to eradicate prostate cancer, according to professionals close to the successful marketing phenomenon.

The Da Vinci System is a big investment, costing $1.5 million, plus a service contract estimated to cost around $150,000 annually. There is also the financial investment of time in training a surgical team. Once the commitment is made, there is no going back, which is why the robot is being billed as the best thing since, well, a radical prostatectomy. The sales pitch has raised some eyebrows. Though the procedure is less traumatic on the body — an undisputed big plus for the patient — the jury is still out on how precise it is at reaching the long-term goal of preventing the cancer from coming back. The surgery just hasn't been in use long enough to collect the data.

The procedure is also not without controversy. The main issue concerns the robot itself. As with the laser-guided technique, robotic surgery lacks a surgeon's important sense of feel. This has raised concern that using robotic arms could cause surgeons to miss some cancer and put patients at a higher risk of cancer recurrence. However, a new study reported in the *British Journal of Urology International* claims this concern is unwarranted. Physician-scientists at New York-Presbyterian Hospital/Weill Cornell Medical Center, using videotapes of more than 1,300 Da Vinci surgeries, demonstrated that the robot, in its own way, has a sense of feel, too.

"Anatomical details and visual cues available through robotic surgery not only allow experienced surgeons to compensate for a lack of tactile feedback, but actually give the illusion of that sensation," says Ashutosh Tewari, M.D., an oncologist who specializes in prostate cancer and the lead author of the study. He said the three-dimensional, high-definition view a surgeon gets while behind the remote console gives the sensation of touch, a phenomenon called intersensory integration. The enhanced vision allowed by the robotic approach brings about "a reverse Braille phenomenon," or the ability for the surgeon to "feel" when vision is enhanced, explained Dr. Tewari.

Robotic surgery is proving itself in other ways. Studies coming out of medical centers that perform a high volume of robotic prostatectomies show that the surgery results in less blood loss and no need for blood transfusions, shorter hospitalization and catheterization, reduced pain, and a faster recovery time than traditional open surgery.

While some centers claim faster recovery of sexual function and urinary control, most independent studies show the rates of impotence and incontinence are just about the same. For example, the Mayo Clinic reported in 2009 that one year after surgery, 30 percent of the men who underwent robotic surgery were impotent and 8 percent were incontinent compared to 40 percent who were impotent and 6 percent who were incontinent one year after undergoing an open nerve-sparing radical prostatectomy.

Studies on its long-term effect are beginning to unfold. Reports from five major medical centers involving nearly 16,500 men found a recurrence rate similar to open surgery after five years. For low-risk disease, the recurrence rate ranged from 6 to 22 percent; for intermediate-risk disease, the recurrence rate ranged from 21 to 37 percent; and for high-risk disease it was 32 to 45 percent. Note that these recurrence rates are far from the "ultimate cure" designation surgeons bestow on robotic surgery's close cousin, manual radical prostatectomy.

Another study investigated robotic surgery as the best option for men interested in continuing their sex life after surgery. One year after performing about 1,000 robotic prostatectomies on men ranging in age from 38 to 85, doctors at the University of Chicago Medical Center found about 69 percent were continent and 75 percent were able to perform sexually.

Despite all the hype and excitement about robotic surgery, there are a lot of doctors who would hesitate to make it their own treatment of choice if they themselves were faced with prostate cancer. Kansas University Medical Center, which offers the surgery, asked a large group of urologists which way they'd go if they had to choose between robotic or a radical prostatectomy. For low-risk disease, a slight majority — 54 percent — said they'd choose robotic surgery. However, if they had high-risk prostate cancer, 59 percent said they'd go the traditional route. The reason? Better tactile sensation, an easier operation for a surgeon to perform, and the scarcity of long-term data on the robot's ability to prevent the cancer from recurring.

Likewise, potential patients should give it careful consideration. Researchers at Duke University Medical Center found that men who opted for robotic laparoscopic surgery were "more likely to be regretful and dissatisfied, possibly because of higher expectation of an 'innovative' procedure."

Big advances in radiation therapy: a better alternative to prostate removal

The results surgeons achieve with prostate surgery have not changed much over the last 10 to 15 years, even with robotic surgery. The story with radiation, however, is different and the methods appear to be ever-improving. Years ago the cure rates with radiation were lower than with surgery and the side effects were worse. Harmful burns to neighboring organs were not uncommon.

Ten years ago, improvements in technology that limited collateral damage put radiation on a par with surgery. Today, however, some radiation therapies have cure rates better than are currently being achieved with surgery and the side effects of radiation are considerably less severe. Advances in technology mean doctors are now able to target and kill cancer cells with precision without risk to other organs. Radiation burns, once a major concern, are almost unheard of today.

Properly targeted, high-dose radiation can often conquer prostate cancer, studies show. The reason? Leaving undetected cancer cells behind is much less likely with radiation. When cutting, surgeons must go out of the border of the malignancy to ensure getting all the cancer. Because the prostate is in a confined space so close to the bladder and rectum, surgeons are only able to obtain a few millimeters of clearance around the gland when they remove it. This means there is a possibility that small amounts of cancer can be left behind. With radiation, the field extends slightly outside the capsule of the prostate gland, which greatly helps ensure against the possibility of cancer spreading. This makes radiation an alluring option for a lot of men.

Radiation therapy uses high-energy X-rays to kill cancer cells. There are two forms of delivery. It can be directed at the body, called external radiation, or it can come from tiny radioactive seeds placed inside the prostate, a method known as brachytherapy.

External beam radiation: zap therapy

The prostate is a very mobile and malleable organ. Even if you're sitting perfectly still, the prostate moves on the will of the bladder or rectum. Any voluntary or involuntary change in these organs can nudge the prostate a tad in one direction or another. This doesn't normally pose a problem, but it can be risky business when a beam of radiation is aimed at a potentially moving target.

In days gone by, radiation posed a considerable threat to a patient because it passes through other organs, such as the rectum or bladder on its way to its target. If a beam misses the prostate even by a few millimeters, it can hit a healthy neighboring organ. The consequences are potentially devastating. If radiation hits healthy intestines it can cause a medley of chronic symptoms including cramping, diarrhea, and constipation — that mimic the symptoms of irritable bowel syndrome. Radiation burns to the rectum can cause chronic proctitis, inflammation of the rectum. This can lead to uncontrollable bowel problems and threaten men with permanent fecal incontinence. It's no wonder that surgery seemed like a much more attractive option!

Fortunately, thanks to advances in radiation technology, these types of threats are not common today, making external radiation a viable treatment option for prostate cancer. Radiation oncologists have made a number of refinements in external beam treatment that can zero in on a subtly moving target without loosing its aim. These advances include three-dimensional conformal radiation therapy (3D-CRT) and the newer generation intensity modulated radiation therapy (IMRT). Now, in addition to eradicating cancerous prostate cells, state-of-the-art external beam therapy helps protect neighboring organs from damage. With the new methods, the risk of severe damage to other organs is only about 2 percent.

In 3D-CRT and IMRT, technicians use CT scans or MRI imaging to create a pattern of the prostate and cancer cells individualized to the patient. Treatment takes place in a special lead-lined room dominated by a giant piece of equipment that aims hundreds of tiny radiation beams of varying intensity at your crotch. You lie on a table in a cradle-like sling made to hold your hips in exact position to keep you from squirming. The beam shape changes hundreds of times during each treatment and can bend around and away from healthy tissue in ways not possible in the past. The treatments are painless but have a few immediate side effects, including fatigue, dry skin and hair loss in the pelvic region, and possibly some diarrhea and urination problems.

The downside of the therapy is that it requires treatment five times a week for seven or eight weeks, and it is not universally available throughout the United States. It could mean extended relocation during the period of therapy and an investment of time and money. Clinics that offer IMRT, however, often also have housing facilities for out-of-town patients. On the upside, doctors encourage men to stay active while getting the treatment. These sophisticated treatments are offered at major centers located in many popular destinations around the country, making a nice spot for a medical tourist to do a little vacationing. For example, Sloan-Kettering Cancer Center, which pioneered IMRT therapy, is located in New York City.

Side effects of radiation therapy

Side effects are part of the program with radiation treatments, just as they are with all prostate cancer procedures. The most immediate symptoms are urinary difficulties. Studies show about 50 percent of men undergoing any form of radiation therapy will experience lower urinary tract symptoms, such as frequent urination, burning during urination, and interruption of sleep due to the need to go to the bathroom. They will generally go away on their own in a few weeks or months.

External beam radiation causes gastrointestinal upsets, though this is more common with 3D-CRT than IMRT.

The risk of long-term urinary problems is about 8 percent and the risk of developing long-term problems as a result of radiation burns to the rectum is about 3 percent.

Problems with erectile dysfunction are slow to develop. An analysis from the Prostate Cancer Outcomes study found 63 percent of men who had radiation therapy complained of erectile dysfunction five years after treatment. Generally, younger men who undergo treatment will maintain the same sexual function after therapy as they had before therapy.

Proton beam radiation: the nuclear reaction

Proton beam radiation is delivered in a manner similar to 3D-CRT and IMRT, but it uses fast-moving, positively charged nuclear subatomic particles, or protons, to kill cancer. The main advantage of protons, according to proponents of the treatment, is that the precision of the proton beam and control of the dosage delivered to the tumor causes minimal damage to surrounding tissue as it passes through on its way to the cancer. With a proton beam, higher doses of radiation can be used to more effectively kill cancer cells, reducing the chance that they could someday come back. Conversely, a lower dose radiation can further reduce the harm to other organs and the consequences that go with it.

Proton beam radiation doesn't get a lot of notice because it is expensive and only about a dozen hospitals in the United States offer it. Though a few more clinics are being planned, it will be slow to grow because of economics. Building a facility involves an investment of $200 million or more. Whether or not it is worth the investment — meaning the quality of life it offers after prostate cancer treatment — is murky. Of the few studies conducted on proton beam therapy and prostate cancer, there is "no proof that it is superior to its alternatives," says Anthony L. Zietman, M.D. An objective statement, considering that Dr. Zietman is a radiation oncologist at Massachusetts General Hospital, one of the U.S. hospitals that offers proton radiation therapy.

The most favorable report to date, according to the National Association for Proton Therapy, comes out of the Proton Treatment Center at Loma Linda University Medical Center in Southern California, which was the first center to bring the therapy to the United States. The study found the overall survival rate for men at all stages of prostate cancer was 89 percent. The study was published in the *International Journal of Radiation Oncology*.

"This is very promising news for prostate cancer patients and shows that we now have a treatment modality that compares favorably, with less side effects, with surgery or traditional radiation treatment," reported the association.

Proton beam therapy is nothing new. It's been in use in Europe and other parts of the world for 40 years, but it didn't appear in the United States until Loma Linda opened its facility in 1990.

Where you can find proton beams

These are the centers in the United States that have a proton beam facility to treat prostate cancer, as well as other forms of the disease:

California (Loma Linda): James M. Slater, M.D. Proton Treatment and Research Center at Loma Linda University Medical Center

Florida (Jacksonville): The University of Florida Proton Therapy Institute

Illinois (Warrington): CDH Proton Center

Illinois (West Chicago): Northern Illinois University Proton Therapy Center

Indiana (Bloomington): Midwest Proton Radiotherapy Institute at Indiana University

Massachusetts (Boston): Francis H. Burr Proton Center at Massachusetts General Hospital

New Jersey (Somerset): ProCure Proton Therapy Center

Oklahoma (Oklahoma City): ProCure Proton Therapy Center at the INTEGRIS Cancer Campus at the University of Oklahoma

Pennsylvania (Philadelphia): The Roberts Proton Therapy Center at the University of Pennsylvania Health System Hampton University Proton Therapy Institute

Texas (Houston): MD Anderson Cancer Center's Proton Center at the University of Texas

Brachytherapy:
highest cure rate, least side effects

Brachytherapy has been around for decades but it really came into its own in the 1990s when doctors perfected the method of delivering high doses of radioactive seeds to cancerous prostate glands with the precision of a heat-seeking missile.

Studies show that brachytherapy has a long-term cure equal to or even better than radical prostatectomy and that it produces "substantially better results" than conventional external beam therapy. It also offers several advantages over these therapies. Compared to prostatectomy:

- there are no incisions and bleeding is generally not worthy of notice.

- the procedure is done on an outpatient basis. You'll be in and out of the hospital in about three hours.

- recovery is rapid — men are back resuming life as usual within 24 to 48 hours.

- brachytherapy offers the best chance of maintaining sexual potency. Studies show that, after surgery, men under age 60 generally maintain the same sexual ability they had before surgery. The rate of diminished sexual ability in older men is about 20 percent.

- urinary complaints are common, but generally minor and short-lived. Most men experience some degree of urinary tract irritation or discomfort, such as frequent urination and burning that lasts for a couple of weeks to a few months.

Unlike external beam therapy, brachytherapy:

- is a once-and-done procedure.

- does not pass radiation through neighboring organs, allowing for a stronger, more effective, dose of radiation where the cancer is.

■ is better able to localize a high dose of radiation within the gland while minimizing the dose outside the gland.

Quality of life: seeds are No. 1

When it comes to restoring quality of life, your best bet is brachytherapy. At least that was the conclusion of the largest study ever conducted on the quality of life outcomes for four different types of invasive treatments for prostate cancer: brachytherapy, open radical prostatectomy, robot-assisted prostatectomy, and cryotherapy.

Brachytherapy was five times better at restoring sexual function and satisfaction than both types of prostatectomy. Cryotherapy had the poorest results. Interestingly, nerve-sparing surgery didn't produce any better overall quality of life results than radical prostatectomy. Brachytherapy and cryotherapy were better than either prostatectomy procedure in restoring urinary control.

The study, based on self-assessment questionnaires, was published in *The Journal of Urology*.

So, if brachytherapy is all it appears to be, why aren't more men opting for it? Many urologists simply aren't offering brachytherapy to their patients as a viable option, says Gordon L. Grado, M.D., founder and medical director of Southwest Oncology Centers based in Phoenix. Most of the patients who end up at one of his four Southwest centers come for a second opinion or as a referral from another patient who had the procedure. When they see how the therapy measures up to surgery, most men want the seed implants.

"For patients, it is much more desirable to spend only three hours in an outpatient surgical center for a seed implantation than to undergo major abdominal or perineal surgery requiring weeks of recovery, or similarly, to submit to protracted daily radiation treatments lasting several weeks," says Dr. Grado.

As cancer treatments go, patients undergoing brachytherapy say it is relatively benign. In the procedure, the surgeon uses needles to direct minute biocompatible titanium cylinders containing radioactive seeds the size of a grain of salt into the prostate in a specific pre-planned pattern that targets the cancer and covers the entire prostate without disturbing the nerves. Anywhere from 80 to 180 seeds are implanted, depending on the size of the prostate. The needles reach the prostate through the perineum, the area between the scrotum and rectum. Proper spacing of the seeds is crucial, as poor spacing means there is potential to miss cancer. The pattern is individualized to each person undergoing the procedure.

Beam, seeds, or both?

It depends on the risk category of your cancer. The general rule of thumb is men with high-risk cancer may be better off with a combination of IMRT and seeds because IMRT can be administered to a slightly broader field, creating a bigger margin around the gland. Adding seeds to IMRT intensifies the radiation dose inside the gland.

For high-risk cancer that has invaded the seminal vesicles, full-dose IMRT is recommended because there currently is no evidence that implanting seeds in the seminal vesicles is effective. For men with cancer that has spread outside the capsule, full-dose IMRT plus seeds is recommended.

IMRT is also recommended for disease that has spread to the lymph nodes — now more rare due to PSA screening.

With brachytherapy, the radiation does not have to pass through other organs, such as the bladder and rectum, to hit its target. The precision and conformation of the procedure enables doctors to deliver a radioactive dose roughly 50 to 100 percent greater than can be safely delivered by conventional external beam therapy, says Dr. Grado. "This is especially important, as increasing evidence shows that local tumor control improves with the amount of radiation delivered."

The cylinders are guided into position by an ultrasound probe that is inserted in the rectum and gives the surgeon a multi-dimensional view of the prostate gland on several television screens. The seeds emit slow doses of declining amounts of radiation, which lasts from three months to a year depending on which type of rapidly decaying radioactive seed is used. The cylinders harmlessly remain in the prostate after the radiation is released.

At the end of the procedure, a catheter is placed in the bladder. It is removed before you leave the recovery room. The procedure is performed under general anesthesia and takes about 45 minutes.

You'll leave the hospital with a short course of antibiotics as a precaution against infection and pain-killing medication, though many men do not find the discomfort after surgery severe enough to take the drugs. The most immediate side effect can be pain and discomfort in the perineum where the needles were inserted.

Brachytherapy as a single therapy is not for everyone. The best candidates for the procedure are men with low-risk cancer and cancer that has advanced and spread throughout the gland but has not escaped the capsule. This would be a man with a Gleason score of 7 or less and a PSA of 10 or less. A combination of seeds and external beam radiation is recommended for men with more advanced cancer. Men at highest risk may benefit from a combination of seeds and hormone therapy.

Men with large prostates generally must go through a course of hormone therapy to shrink the prostate before the procedure can be performed.

Surgery versus brachytherapy: what the studies say

When researchers analyze cure rates, they look at two things: the quality of the treatment and the average risk. Two prestigious institutions — Johns Hopkins University Medical Center in Baltimore, Maryland and The Prostate Cancer Treatment Center in Seattle, Washington — each did their own independent analysis of the outcomes of radical surgery and seed implantation over the course of 15 years.

Johns Hopkins, reporting in the journal *Urology*, found the cure rate for surgery was 85 percent in low-risk patients, 63 percent in men who were intermediate-risk, and 40 percent in high-risk disease. Seattle's Prostate Treatment Center published their results at about the same time in the *International Journal of Radiation Oncology* and found the cure rate for seed implantation was 86 percent for low-risk disease, 80 percent for intermediate-risk cancer, and 68 percent for high-risk disease.

In another study, Peter D. Grimm, D.O. of the Prostate Cancer Treatment Center analyzed the cure rates of 12 U.S. institutions using surgery and 24 using seed implants and seed implants came in first. Here's what he found:

Cancer type	Surgery cure rate	Seed implants cure rate
Low-risk	85%	95%
Medium-risk	70%	85%
High-risk	40%	75%

Not only does brachytherapy offer fewer side effects and complications, it also offers the most promising cure rate!

Some argue that these statistics may be somewhat skewed because men undergoing surgery relapse about five years earlier than men who undergo brachytherapy. But even this is good news! Delaying a relapse by five years in and of itself is a good argument to prefer seeds over surgery.

Blocking male hormones to fight cancer: great in theory, not in practice

Prostate cancer is exquisitely sensitive to the male hormone testosterone. It grows in its presence, and it stops growing and can even regress when testosterone is taken away. The anticancer effects of testosterone deprivation are indisputable. In 1966 the late Charles B. Huggins, M.D., a Canadian-born American urologist, won the Nobel Prize in medicine for his discovery that cancer cells are dependent on chemical signals from substances, such as hormones, to grow and survive.

Back then, the only way to stop testosterone production and prolong the life of men with aggressive prostate cancer was to remove the testicles — what is medically called a bilateral orchiectomy — or to put it bluntly, castration. These days the same effect can be achieved by taking drugs, a treatment option called androgen deprivation therapy, or androgen blockade. The treatment, however, is and always has been controversial.

> Numerous studies over the years have produced disappointing results after depriving prostate cancer of testosterone. Apparently, it is the slow-growing nondeadly types of cancer cells that are most dependent on testosterone for growth. The rare, fast-growing cancer cells don't seem to be much affected by testosterone deprivation. There doesn't seem to be much, if any, benefit, measured by fatalities, but there are lots of problems that occur when testosterone production is suppressed.

Androgen deprivation therapy: putting cancer in remission

The only other cancer that is sensitive to hormone therapy is breast cancer. Take away the female hormone estrogen and certain forms of breast cancer stop growing. Prostate cancer, however, is so hormone sensitive that androgen deprivation therapy is five times more effective at slowing tumor growth than even the best breast cancer therapy. However, this does not mean that hormone therapy is a viable treatment for anything but extreme cases.

Androgen deprivation therapy causes a fast and dramatic drop in testosterone levels, occurring over a matter of weeks. As a result, some cancer cells stop growing and tumors commit cellular suicide, a process called apoptosis.

As effective as it is at stopping testosterone, hormone deprivation therapy traditionally has been reserved as a means to prolong life in men with late-stage cancer that has spread to the lymph nodes, bones, or other sites. As a treatment for early-stage prostate cancer, it is contentious. There are several reasons why most doctors do not consider testosterone deprivation a formidable treatment for early-stage disease, including a devastating and long list of side effects. These are the major conflicts.

It is not a cure. Hormone therapy can only put prostate cancer in remission. Once the therapy is ended, testosterone eventually comes back and so does the cancer.

It can't kill certain cancer cells. Some prostate cancer cells are so virulent they will grow even in the absence of testosterone. This is called androgen-independent prostate cancer. The longevity of a man who chooses androgen deprivation therapy ultimately depends on the cellular composition of his cancer — that is, the ratio of androgen-dependent cells to androgen-independent cells. The greater the number of androgen-dependent cells to androgen-independent cells, the more likely the cancer will respond to hormone therapy.

It doesn't kill all the cancer all the time. Hormone therapy causes detectable nodules to disappear and PSA levels to sharply decline, a sign the therapy seems to be working. However, studies have found it does not eradicate every last prostate cancer cell in the majority of men — especially the most virulent cells.

It increases cholesterol. Studies show hormone therapy increases blood cholesterol. In one study total cholesterol increased an average of 9 percent. Triglycerides, another type of blood fat that increases a man's risk of heart disease, stroke, and diabetes, went up 27 percent. Many experts feel the benefits of the therapy do not outweigh this risk.

It raises the risk of heart trouble. An analysis of two large health databases found that men on hormone therapy were 11 percent more likely to have a heart attack and 16 percent more likely to develop a life-threatening disturbance in heart rhythm that can cause the heart to stop beating.

It decreases the ability to metabolize sugar. The same analysis found men on hormone therapy had a 44 percent increase in the risk of developing diabetes. The drug therapy decreases insulin sensitivity, interfering with the body's ability to respond to insulin, the hormone necessary to remove a type of sugar called glucose from the blood.

It's like chemical castration. A major objection to giving hormone drugs to men with early-stage cancer is what the lack of testosterone does to a man's love life — it destroys it. Men who take testosterone-depleting drugs find their interest in sex comes to a fast and screeching halt. The effect is both physical and emotional. Opponents of the therapy see it as the equivalent of chemical castration.

It causes male menopause. Androgen deprivation therapy produces side effects similar to those a woman experiences going through menopause — hot flashes, night sweats, mood swings, weight gain, and brittle bones. Some men find they can get uncharacteristically emotional. The final indignity is that hormone therapy causes the breasts to enlarge, which occurs because estrogen starts taking over for the lack of testosterone.

It decreases muscle mass and increases fat. Testosterone is what makes rock-hard abs when you exercise. Shutting down testosterone production causes muscle mass to turn into fat. In one study of men who took the therapy for a year, lean muscle mass declined 4 percent and fat mass increased 11 percent.

It accelerates osteoporosis. Older men on hormone therapy have a 57 percent increased risk of multiple fractures associated with osteoporosis, according to an analysis of 46,587 men by researchers at The Cancer Institute of New Jersey.

It increases the risk of colon cancer. An analysis of more than 107,000 men found the risk of colon cancer was 30 to 40 percent higher in men who took hormone therapy for prostate cancer than in men who didn't take the therapy. The risk increased with the length of time on the therapy.

The good new is that, for most men, these side effects are reversible. Virtually all the side effects will eventually go away after the therapy is stopped. Some oncologists feel it is an argument for at least giving it a try, which in itself makes it an attractive option. Unlike other therapies, if a man can't deal with the side effects of the drugs, the treatment can be stopped with no permanent damage. However, shrinkage of the prostate gland after therapy may preclude or interfere with surgery, should that be necessary in the future. Otherwise, life goes back to the way it was and he can find another way to deal with his cancer.

Not tonight, I have a ...

As with other types of prostate cancer therapy, testosterone deprivation does a number on your sex life, but in the case of hormone therapy, it does it big time. And it has nothing to do with the inability to get an erection. In a matter of days after starting hormone therapy, interest in sex is history. Libido is zapped. Your hot buttons freeze. Whatever aroused you before now leaves you limp. Erectile dysfunction becomes a moot point when you have no libido. Many men find the feeling to be so unnatural it is disturbing.

Loss of libido and sexual dysfunction are part of the package for 90 percent of men taking androgen replacement therapy. When the therapy is stopped, they don't automatically return either. It takes time, and how long it takes depends on your age, the type and length of hormone treatment, your general health, and your emotional stamina. Most men will recover libido and potency within a few months; for others it can take up to a year. Even after testosterone returns, 25 percent of men over age 65 say their libido is permanently flagged.

And now, the good news about hormone therapy

There is no consensus among experts as to when or if a man with prostate cancer should consider hormone therapy. The traditional view is that it should be reserved only for late-stage prostate cancer that has spread to the bones. There is a less popular school of thought that supports it for less-entrenched, early-stage cancer. One such proponent is Mark Scholz, M.D., a Southern California oncologist who specializes in prostate cancer and is the author of the book *Invasion of the Prostate Snatchers.*

The primary reason hormone therapy is not a popular option for early-stage cancer is the reality that the disease eventually resurfaces. Also, cancer cells can grow a resistance to the medication. "The medical community has wrongly assumed that remission in men with early-stage disease will be just as brief as in men with bone metastasis, lasting only three to six years," Dr. Scholz writes in his book.

According to studies conducted by Dr. Scholz, men who start the therapy before cancer has a chance to spread beyond the prostate can keep the disease in remission for more than 10 years before the body develops a resistance to the therapy. Even if the disease is not arrested, he says, it delays progression for many years.

In one study, reported in the journal *Oncology*, more than 95 percent of men with newly diagnosed disease saw a drop in their PSA to less than 0.05 within eight months of therapy. This is not necessarily a sure sign that the disease has been arrested in its most virulent form. If hormone therapy does not cause PSA to fall within a safe threshold or PSA starts to rise, Dr. Scholz recommends additional treatment with radiation.

Proponents support androgen deprivation for low-risk prostate cancer for reasons that primarily have to do with maintaining quality of life. There is no risk of lifelong impotence and incontinence, the main objection to radical prostatectomy. Plus, all the other risks and possible complications associated with surgery and radiation treatments are avoided. And while the side effects of androgen therapy are severe, supporters argue that they can be controlled through diligent lifestyle practices. For example:

- Weight gain can be controlled through diet and exercise.
- Loss of muscle mass can be diminished by doing weight-bearing exercise.

- Breast enlargement can be avoided by getting a low dose of radiation prior to treatment or taking the drug letrozole (Femara), which was originally designed to decrease the risk of breast cancer recurrence. In men it has been found to stop the conversion of testosterone to estrogen. This drug, however, carries its own share of potentially severe side effects, the biggest of which is bone loss severe enough to lead to osteoporosis.

- Bone loss can be controlled by taking the drugs bisphosphonate pamidronate (Aredia) and zoledronic acid (Zometa).

- Sildenafil (Viagra) or other erection-enhancing drugs can fill in for the absence of libido.

- If testosterone is too slow to return after therapy is stopped, a topical testosterone gel (AndroGel 1%) can be applied to bring it back.

- Taking an aspirin a day can lower the risk of heart disease and blot clots.

Critics of the therapy for low-risk disease, however, just don't buy it. They see the therapy only as a last-ditch effort to help prolong life in men whose disease has spread. Because the therapy offers no solution to long-term control of cancer, they say it shouldn't be an option for men with low-risk disease. They caution that careful consideration should be given to the impact of the severe side effects on your life.

How hormone therapy works

Hormone therapy works by blocking the testosterone production process that starts in the brain and ends in the prostate. The hypothalamus is the hormone-processing center of the brain. At regular intervals, the hypothalamus signals the neighboring pituitary gland to secrete a substance called luteinizing hormone-releasing hormone (LHRH) that, in turn, signals special cells in the testicles to release testosterone into the bloodstream. An enzyme called 5-alpha-reductase stimulates the conversion of testosterone to dihydrotestosterone

(DHT), the active form primarily responsible for fueling the growth of cells. Hormone deprivation therapy works by interfering with this sequence of events. All the drugs carry most of the significant side effects associated with the therapy.

The ultimate goal — the destruction of cancer cells — is monitored through frequent PSA blood testing. If PSA falls below a level of 4 within three to six months of initiating hormone therapy, it is a sign that the disease is regressing. A PSA nadir — that is, the lowest level reached after treatment — of 0.05 is the best indication that hormone therapy was worth the trouble.

Therapy can include one drug or a combination of drugs, although combination therapy is proving to be more effective. The drugs can be taken continuously to keep testosterone out of production or by a method called intermittent androgen suppression. In this fashion, the drugs are used until testosterone and PSA levels drop and then discontinued. They only come into play again when PSA levels start to rise again. Some doctors believe this on-and-off cycle delays the emergence of life-threatening, androgen-resistant cancer cells.

The main testosterone-arresting drugs are generally given as monthly injections in the abdomen. They include two types of drugs that go after LHRH in different ways.

LHRH agonists. Luteinizing hormone-releasing hormone (LHRH) agonists, which also go by the name gonadotropin-releasing hormone (GnRH) agonists, are a type of synthetic drug with the same chemical structure as natural LHRH. They have traditionally been the drug of choice for hormone deprivation therapy.

LHRH agonists work in somewhat of an odd way. Because the brain recognizes the drug as LHRH, it sets in motion the same hormone-producing network as natural LHRH, only it exaggerates it. After a short time, however, the brain senses something "different" and reverses course, turning off hormone production. It generally takes about two to three weeks for this to happen.

In the meantime, the initial stoking of testosterone can have a troublesome impact on some men, especially those whose cancer has already spread. To prevent this, doctors often prescribe an antiandrogen receptor bicalutamide (Casodex) that prevents testosterone from stimulating cancer cells. It is taken until testosterone is arrested and levels start to fall.

The LHRH agonist most commonly used is leuprolide (Lupron). In addition to injection, leuprolide can also be implanted under the skin as a time-release medication that lasts for a year. Other forms of injectable LHRH agonists are goserelin (Zoladex) and triptorelin (Trelstar).

LHRH antagonists. This group of drugs, also known as GnRH receptor antagonists, hit the scene in 2008. The advantage is that these drugs don't cause an initial increase in testosterone before they get to work.

LHRH antagonists work on the molecular level by deactivating luteinizing hormone receptors in the pituitary gland, thus preventing the testicles from producing testosterone. Studies show that it is as effective as leuprolide in reducing testosterone levels. The drug goes by the name degarelix (Firmagon).

Antiandrogen receptors. These drugs can play an important role in hormone therapy because their primary job is to prevent testosterone from binding to and stimulating cancer cells. Testosterone's rendezvous with cancer cells takes place in a special spot called androgen receptor sites. Antiandrogen receptors break up this unhealthy union by getting to and by occupying the site first.

Antiandrogen receptors make a helpful addition to hormone therapy, but they are seldom used alone because they may not be sufficient. They don't stop testosterone production, the primary goal of hormone therapy. Because they aren't involved in testosterone production, antiandrogen receptors are the least likely among the hormone therapy drugs to interfere with a man's sex life, but they do carry most of the other untoward side effects.

In addition to bicalutamide, antiandrogen receptors are also marketed as flutamid and nilutamide (Niladron).

Synthetic estrogen: the debate continues

The forerunner to LHRH agonists was the synthetic form of the female hormone estrogen called Premarin that could lower testosterone as effectively as surgical castration. The drug carries a high risk of heart attack, stroke, and blood clots and fell out of favor as a testosterone-killing drug when the U.S. Food and Drug Administration approved LHRH agonists.

There is now a renewed interest in using another form of estrogen called diethylstilbestrol (DES) for men with advanced disease. DES was widely used in the 1960s to help prevent miscarriages until it was discovered that it could cause fertility problems in men and women whose mother had taken the drug.

Surgical castration: the path of most resistance

As difficult as it may be to imagine, medical castration is still used today in men whose cancer has grown out of control. The reason? It is the most effective and least expensive way to stop testosterone production. Unlike with drug therapy, the benefit is immediate. Testosterone drops to what doctors call castrate level within 12 hours. The side effects — the same experienced with drug therapy — are also immediate.

As surgery goes, and in comparison to a prostatectomy, surgical castration is considered relatively easy — to the surgeon. The procedure takes about 20 minutes under anesthesia on an outpatient basis. Neither the operation nor the recovery is considered to be painful.

The procedure involves making a small incision in the scrotum and removing each testicle. You can also opt to have only the contents of the testicles removed and leave the shell in place. It is said to make for a more normal outward appearance.

Though it is the most effective way to stop testosterone production, only about a quarter of men faced with life-threatening prostate cancer undergo the procedure. For many men, the idea of castration is too emotionally devastating to even consider.

Alternative treatments: going to extremes

There are times when desperation calls for desperate measures, but one of those times should not be when you have cancer. For decades, shady opportunists and poorly conducted research have pushed dozens of unfounded treatments — shark cartilage and potentially poisonous apricot pits the most notorious among them.

Alternative treatments, however, are different from unfounded treatments, and two in particular are proving to measure up to scientific scrutiny. They literally take killing cancer to extremes. One freezes it and the other fries it. Both have been called a viable alternative option for men desiring a treatment somewhere between hands-off active surveillance and radical surgery.

Cryoablation surgery: freeze therapy

Cryo means cold. Ablation means excision. Cryoablation means freezing cancer to death.

Also known by the moniker ice ball therapy, the procedure involves filling the prostate with liquid nitrogen at an exceptionally low temperature to kill cancer while protecting neighboring organs with warm circulating saline solution.

In the procedure, the surgeon first inserts a warming coil filled with saline solution into the urethra and bladder to protect the organs from the deep freeze. He then inserts thin needles called cryoprobes through the perineum and into the prostate. An ultrasound probe is inserted into the rectum to guide the placement of the needles.

Once inserted, freezing gas drops the temperature of the cryoprobes to around minus 40 degrees. The low temperature creates ice balls that freeze the entire prostate and some of the nearby tissue. After the prostate is frozen, it is thawed and the freeze-thaw cycle is repeated a second time to reduce the chance that any cancerous cells are still alive.

The procedure is performed under anesthesia and takes from two to three hours. You'll usually remain in the hospital overnight and wear a catheter for about two weeks.

Cryosurgery is hardly new. It's been in use for more than 40 years, but has always been considered salvage therapy reserved for men whose cancer has recurred after receiving radiation. Today, however, it has risen to a new level of interest as better technology has made the procedure safer and more effective.

The five-year survival rates for early-stage and late-stage prostate cancer treated with ice ball therapy are comparable to radical prostatectomy, according to Fletcher Derrick, M.D., who has been performing the procedure at Roper Hospital of the Medical University of South Carolina in Charleston since 1999. He reports survival rates ranging from 60 to 92 percent for early-stage cancer and 36 to 89 percent for high-risk cancer.

Doctors speculate that the wide range in the five-year success rate may have to do with the potential for leaving cancer behind. The warming coil that protects the urethra and bladder also protects a minute degree of surrounding tissue, meaning if residual cancer exists in this tissue, it will remain behind. The surgery carries these risks and side effects:

- swelling of the prostate, penis, and scrotum following surgery

- numbness in the penis that can last up to four months

- a 93 percent certainty of impotence

- urethral sloughing in about 15 percent of men who under- take the procedure; this is a condition in which dead tissue passes through the urethra, and can potentially obstruct urine flow

■ a 2 to 4 percent risk of incontinence

Cryosurgery is not widely used as a treatment, because outcomes are not generally as good as with other therapies.

Nomograms: the new cool tool

You can do a do-it-yourself projection of the optimal outcome of prostate cancer before and after treatment through an easy-to-access Internet tool created by doctors at Memorial Sloan-Kettering Cancer Center in New York City.

The tool, called nomograms, is available to doctors to help them determine the best treatment for their patients, but men with prostate cancer are welcome to use it, too. All you need to do is log on to *www.nomograms.org*, click on "prostate cancer" and follow the directions. To do your self-assessment you will need to know a few things about your cancer, such as your Gleason score, your PSA level, and tumor size, all of which are available from your doctor.

The site is intended to be used only as a guide and to help men work with their doctor to guide treatment options.

High-intensity focused ultrasound: heat therapy

Scientists are starting to give cautious but promising high fives to HIFU, the acronym for High-Intensity Focused Ultrasound, the "tropical" alternative to freezing cryoablation.

Its claim to fame is what it offers a man in terms of quality of life: no loss of potency. Researchers in Great Britain report there is no loss of sexual function in 80 to 90 percent of men having the procedure, making it a big advantage over most other treatments, with the possible exception of brachytherapy that is a close second. By treating the tumor rather than the whole prostate, side effects across the board are minimized. There is no incision, so it sidesteps the infection rate and other risks associated with surgery.

In the procedure, a dual-action wand is inserted into the rectum next to the prostate to locate the cancer and divide the gland into treatment zones. The surgeon then uses a high-energy beam that raises the temperature of the cancer site or sites to the near boiling temperature of 194 degrees in a matter of seconds. The beam essentially cooks the cancer. The procedure takes about 20 minutes on an outpatient basis. A catheter will be in place for about two weeks. Side effects include:

- urinary difficulties, particularly a slow stream, that can last for several months.

- swelling of the prostate that lasts for several months.

- urethral sloughing, which can impede urine flow.

HIFU has been in popular use in Europe since 1998 but the U.S. FDA has not yet approved it and it is only being used on an experimental basis in the United States. One of the handful of treatment centers in the United States that is experimenting with the treatment is the University of Texas MD Anderson Cancer Center in Houston, Texas. "This therapy has been used in Europe to treat 17,000 men with various stages of prostate cancer, and from that experience it appears to be a promising balance between effective cancer treatment and few long-term effects," says John Ward, M.D., assistant professor of Anderson's Department of Urology.

Nevertheless, long-term data is limited but studies have found that 70 percent of men with low- and intermediate-risk diseases were still cancer-free after five years.

The organization International HIFU, which is located in Charlotte, N.C., can help guide you to treatment centers in Canada, Mexico, Bermuda, the Caribbean, South America, India, and Europe. For more information on doctors who perform the procedure and treatment centers go to *www.internationalhifu.com*.

Want to experiment?

If you want to experiment with prostate cancer treatment, think twice because you are trading an option to get a proven treatment for something unproven. However, if you're interested in trying new things, your best bet is to participate in research and become part of a clinical trial — a research study which experiments on humans.

Researchers use clinical trials to find out if promising new treatment methods are safe and really work. At the end of the study, the data is collected and printed in a medical journal. Eventually, if a treatment proves successful, it will be given approval by the U.S. Food and Drug Administration.

Trials can compare a new experimental treatment against another — usually the method that has been around the longest and for which the most data has accumulated, what scientists call the gold standard. For example, radical prostatectomy is the gold standard for prostate cancer treatment. The downside of getting in such a research study is that you may be assigned to a specific treatment randomly, meaning you don't get a choice.

Studies on drugs do the same — measure the effectiveness of an experimental drug against the gold standard. Sometimes the test drug is measured against a placebo, a sugar pill. This, too, is frequently a randomized study.

If you become part of a trial, the study's sponsor should cover all the medical costs related to the experiment. To qualify for a clinical trial, you will have to match a specific set of criteria.

All the clinical studies being conducted on prostate cancer can be found on the National Institutes of Health's website, *www.clinical trials.gov*.

Comparing treatments

Treatments for prostate cancer are frequently compared from two points of view. One considers quality of life — the risk of ending up with long-term problems involving impotence and incontinence. The other considers long-term survival, the ultimate judge of a treatment's effectiveness.

These three charts show the range of rates a select group of studies have found for incontinence, impotence, and survival for popular treatment options. The survival-rate chart is based on a percentage rate five years after treatment.

Treatment	Incontinence rate
HIFU	0-2%
Brachytherapy	1-7%
External beam radiation	0-15%
Prostatectomy	0-19%
Cryotherapy	7-52%

Treatment	Impotence rate
HIFU	10-30%
Brachytherapy	14-40%
External beam radiation	50-61%
Prostatectomy	14-90%
Cryotherapy	47-95%

Treatment	Low-risk disease survival rate	Intermediate-risk disease survival rate
HIFU	70-71%	70-71%
Brachytherapy	78-89%	66-82%
External beam radiation	81-86%	26-60%
Prostatectomy	76-98%	37-77%
Cryotherapy	60-92%	61-89%

PSA rising: advanced disease and what it means

Sadly, prostate cancer remains a killer. About 24,000 men die each year from the disease, even though it is rare these days to discover the disease in a late stage. Prostate cancer is second only to lung cancer as the leading cause of cancer death among American men.

So if the disease is being caught so early and is so slow-growing, why is it considered such a major cancer threat? Several factors come into play.

Cancer cells play hide and seek. With all the advances in treatment methods, doctors cannot know for sure if all traces of cancer cells are excised along with the tumor, no matter what treatment is being used. Surgeons are particularly handicapped because the prostate is so small. For example, a small piece of the prostate is left behind in surgery in order to attach the urethra to the bladder. In cryotherapy, a margin of tissue surrounding the urethra is left unharmed in order not to damage the organ. If undetected cancer exists in the tissue, the cancer can continue to grow.

Metastatic disease is hard to beat. Some men simply are at high risk of their cancer spreading — a deceptive gene that spawns rare but virulent cancer cells that resist treatment and begin to spread. The most troublesome form of the disease is called androgen-resistant disease. It grows even when the cancer's main fuel, testosterone, is shut down.

Men get a feeling of false security. Even if you've had the so-called ultimate treatment, a radical prostatectomy, there is no telling in the long run that it has cured *you*. Being a cancer survivor means you must be forever vigilant. For a man with prostate disease, it means getting a digital rectal exam and a PSA blood test yearly — or twice yearly, if that's what your doctor wants. A rising PSA is a warning sign the disease is coming back. Prostate cancer death statistics are filled with men who stopped following up on their disease.

The first two factors you can do little about. The third is totally within your power to control.

Life in the comfort zone

No matter how high your PSA was before treatment, it's going to take a dramatic drop after treatment. It's the key indicator that what you've gone through was worth the effort.

Even though the PSA test becomes a house of cards for men with detectable disease that never would have been a problem in their lifetime, the blood test is a lifeline for men after treatment. In fact, the PSA test was originally designed to probe for recurrence of cancer after surgery, not as a diagnostic tool.

After surgery or radiation, doctors want to see a PSA reading that is virtually undetectable. This is a good sign that all malignancy has been removed. It can rise after that, but a PSA under 0.05 is considered to be in the comfort zone — a sign the disease has been contained — though this can vary depending on the kind of treatment you had. A PSA that stays steady as the years advance is a significant sign that you aren't going to die from prostate cancer. On the other hand, men whose PSA doubles within three months of treatment are at the highest risk for dying from the disease.

If PSA doesn't take a dramatic nosedive following surgery, it is an indication that undetectable cancer had already escaped the capsule even before surgery. What doctors watch out for during the years after surgery is what they call PSA doubling time — the amount of time it takes for PSA to go from say a 2 to a 4. If PSA levels start to rise a few months or even years after surgery, and continue to rise, it means all the cancer was not caught. In essence, you've got it again. Doctors call this biochemical failure. The American Society of Therapeutic Radiology and Oncology defines biochemical failure as three consecutive increases in PSA measured six months apart.

If this happens, it is not necessarily a cause for panic. Even if the disease comes back, it's possible it can be arrested as long as it is detected in time — the reason why you don't want to miss a follow-up appointment with your doctor. The consensus among experts is that a PSA of 4 or below in cases of biochemical recurrence, is treatable. External beam radiation is usually the first line of defense after biochemical failure.

Remember, prostate cancer is slow-growing. A rapidly growing recurrence does happen, but it is rare. More likely, if the cancer is going to come back, it is going to take years to develop. This is why scientists keep track of men who've been treated for the disease for 10, 12, or even 15 years. The risk of residual cancer showing up as a rising PSA 10 years after surgery in men who had been treated for early-stage cancer is around 30 percent, according to statistics.

Be careful of word mincing

Watchful waiting and active surveillance are frequently used interchangeably as a nontreatment approach to dealing with many diseases. In cancer, however, watchful waiting can mean something different: forgoing treatment because the prognosis for the disease does not look good, whether treated or not.

With active surveillance, treatment is put off until a time when or if it is necessary. However, when disease progresses under the designation of watchful waiting, doctors move on to what they call palliative treatment, meaning therapy aimed at relieving pain and limiting complications rather than trying to cure the disease. Watchful waiting in prostate cancer is an option put on the table for men with advanced disease.

Palliative treatments can include a procedure called transurethral resection of the prostate (TURP), a popular treatment for men with benign prostatic hyperplasia to relieve urinary symptoms; hormone deprivation therapy; or radiation for disease that has spread to other organs.

Men with advanced disease opting for watchful waiting should contact their doctor at the first sign of urinary difficulties, blood in the urine, or pelvic or back pain.

Managing advancing disease

Some prostate cancer cells are so powerful and dangerous they resist arrest by any treatment. These cells pack a cellular punch akin to a category five hurricane. Scientific attempt to identify prostate cells set on a search-and-destroy mission — and spot them early on — has been like trying to find a needle in a haystack. Most recently, researchers at Weill Cornell Medical College in New York City made a big breakthrough in understanding how prostate cancer cells become lethal when they identified specific genes that fuse and cause cancer cells to mutate into lethal cells. They believe this discovery will lead to finding more individualized therapies to eradicate cells destined to become deadly.

Advanced prostate cancer means the disease has spread beyond the prostate into the seminal vesicles, to the lymph nodes, and to the bones. As yet, there is no cure for prostate cancer that has traveled so far. Treatment is aimed at reducing pain and prolonging life.

The series of events that lead up to advanced prostate cancer begins when PSA takes a big leap. Radiation therapy, if it hasn't failed already, is sometimes used as the first line of defense against recurring disease in men who have had a prostatectomy or other treatments that did not involve radiation. Eventually — and usually sooner rather than later — androgen deprivation therapy is introduced. This can sometimes put cancer in remission for years. The worst cancerous cells, however, are resistant to androgen therapy. This is when other, less effective salvage measures are taken.

Until recently, the treatment of last resort has been chemotherapy, though it isn't as effective against prostate cancer as it can be with other cancers. Ironically, the reason is due to prostate cancer's penchant to grow slowly. You see, chemotherapy cannot discriminate between healthy cells and sick cells. It wants to attack them all, but it starts by going after the fastest-growing cells, which are cancer cells and hair cells. This is why losing hair is a common side effect of chemotherapy. Unfortunately, chemotherapy's ability to extend life for a man with prostate cancer can be counted in months, at best, rather than years. The newest generation of chemotherapy for prostate cancer, and the longest-acting, is the drug docetaxel (Taxotere).

A major breakthrough in treating advanced prostate cancer came in 2010 when the FDA approved a "vaccine" called sipuleucel-T

(Provenge). Although it is called a vaccine, it has nothing to do with preventing disease. Its only target is advanced disease. Studies have found that sipuleucel-T can extend life for men with advanced-stage prostate cancer longer than any chemotherapy drug has been able to achieve.

During experimental studies, researchers found sipuleucel-T extended the lives of men with metastatic androgen-resistant disease by several years, which was four months longer than the best response from any chemotherapy drug.

Another drug still in the early experimental stage, called MDV3100, was found to reduce the number of circulating tumor cells and stabilize advanced disease in a small group of men, according to a study reported in the journal *The Lancet*.

Until science can better understand how prostate cancer becomes lethal, finding a treatment that can effectively beat advanced prostate cancer will continue to be a stab in the dark. In the meantime, the focus will be on trying to extend the longevity and quality of life for men with advanced disease. As of now, approximately 75 percent of men with metastatic disease have a survival rate of five years, 15 percent have a five-to-10 year survival rate, and 10 percent live more than 10 years.

Quality of life: what patients have to say

There is no discussion of prostate cancer treatments that doesn't include these three little words: Quality of life. They come up *a lot*. For many men they create more anguish than the cancer itself.

Medical science has yet to come up with a way of killing prostate cancer without sacrifice in your personal life, at least temporarily. Even choosing no treatment at all, active surveillance, can take a toll. Many men find it hard to handle the knowledge of having cancer in the body and intentionally leaving it alone. For some, it causes anxiety and depression that diminish quality of life.

In the medical arena, quality of life after invasive prostate cancer treatment involves physical limitations and difficulties in three areas: sexual function, urinary problems, and bowel control. Many major treatment centers keep track of the quality of life of its patients for years following treatment through questionnaires it asks them to fill out periodically. The type of questions asked will give you an idea of the challenges many men face as a result of having an invasive treatment procedure. On these questionnaires, men are asked to rank the level of "bother" in these areas.

Sexual problems

- level of sexual desire

- ability to get an erection

- ability and frequency of morning erections

- quality of erection

- ability to have an orgasm

- frequency of sexual activity

Urinary problems

- number of pads worn per day as a result of incontinence

- frequency of urination

- burning sensation while urinating

- weak stream

- uncontrollable leakage (stress incontinence)

- interruption of sleep to urinate

- blood in urine

Bowel problems

- uncontrollable leakage

- loose, watery stools

- painful bowel movements

- bloody stools

- cramping in the abdomen, pelvis, or rectum

Quality of life? Brachytherapy wins!

"Health-related quality of life concerns factor prominently in prostate cancer management," note researchers from the Virginia Prostate Center at Eastern Virginia Medical School in Norfolk, Va., who attempted to figure out which treatment fared best in protecting quality of life in the long run. To find out, they reviewed the questionnaires filled out by nearly 800 men at seven different times over the course of three years, including right before they had their procedure. The treatments they assessed were open radical prostatectomy, the da Vinci robotic-assisted laparoscopic radical prostatectomy, brachytherapy, and cryotherapy.

The winner? Brachytherapy, on all scores. Though all the treatments created quality-of-life issues, they were resolved faster with brachytherapy. Men who had brachytherapy experienced a return to normal sexual function fivefold greater than those who underwent other therapies. Men who received either brachytherapy or cryotherapy had much better overall scores in recovery of urinary control. Bowel problems, if any, generally resolved quickly with all treatments.

From a quality-of-life perspective, the researchers found no difference between the two different types of radical prostatectomy.

Though prostate treatments can create anguish regarding quality of life, it doesn't mean continence and an active love life are a lost cause. There are ways to deal with both, which is what the next chapters are about.

New use for 'tainted' drug

Back in the 1950s a medical scandal of major proportions erupted because what was believed to be a benign over-the-counter sedative that could relieve the symptoms of morning sickness in pregnant women turned out to cause major birth defects. The drug thalidomide was banned from the market, but not before it maimed more than 10,000 children worldwide. It is still considered to be one of the biggest medical tragedies of modern times.

Thalidomide is now back in the news, this time as a promising drug to slow the progression of advancing prostate cancer. Researchers have found the drug interferes with the abnormal growth of blood vessels that feed cancer cells.

The initial experimental stage of a study involving 159 men with prostate cancer found that taking androgen-replacement therapy with thalidomide kept the disease in remission 50 percent longer than taking the therapy along with a placebo — from 10 months to 15 months. A second study found remission lasted even longer — 17 months compared to 10.

Comparing your options

Active surveillance

Advantages	Disadvantages	Ideal candidate
There are no side effects and no threat to your sex life. Treatment can be delayed for years. It's possible you'll never need treatment. Safely delaying treatment means that it's possible better treatment options could become available if or when you need treatment. Long-term risk of death is not elevated compared to immediate treatment.	The anxiety of knowing you have cancer and are not attempting to "cut it out." You'll have to undergo yearly or twice-yearly testing, including some repeat biopsies for the rest of your life.	Any man with low-risk cancer, meaning a Gleason score of less than 7 and a PSA of 4 or less. While some doctors feel the ideal candidates for active surveillance are only older men, this thinking is gradually changing. Many experts believe and studies show this approach is safe for men of all ages.

Androgen deprivation therapy

Advantages	Disadvantages	Ideal candidate
It may prolong life and help reduce pain in cancer that has spread to the bones or other sites, but may not be effective in other cases.	Some older men report sexual interest doesn't completely return with cessation of therapy.	It has traditionally been reserved for men with advanced, high-risk disease.

Advantages	Disadvantages	Ideal candidate
There is no risk of incontinence and the risk of permanent impotence is small. If you have low-risk disease and don't like the side effects, the therapy can be stopped immediately and another treatment chosen.	It is not a cure. Rather it slows down growth in less aggressive cancer cells. Side effects are major, and include: ■ increased risk of death from other diseases ■ breast enlargement ■ loss of libido ■ osteoporosis ■ hot flashes ■ anemia	

Brachytherapy

Advantages	Disadvantages	Ideal candidate
A minimally invasive alternative to radical prostatectomy without many of the risks of complications associated with surgery. Offers the best outcome in terms of quality of life. Cancer cure rate equal to or better than all other treatments. Recovery is generally swift — just a day or two.	Can produce lower urinary tract irritation that lasts from a few weeks to a few months. A very low risk of damage to the rectum, which can result in long-term problems.	A man with early-stage disease or disease throughout the gland that has not escaped the capsule. Men with large prostates may have to undergo hormone therapy to shrink the prostate prior to treatment. Men who have undergone surgical treatment for an enlarged prostate are poor candidates for the procedure.

Comparing your options *continued*

External beam radiation

Advantages	Disadvantages	Ideal candidate
No incision or risks associated with invasive procedures and anesthesia.	The treatment takes place on a daily basis for seven or eight weeks.	All men with prostate cancer are candidates for radiation.
Little or no risk of urinary difficulty.	There is a 2 to 4% risk of rectal burn and long-term complications.	In men with advanced disease, it may be recommended in addition to other treatments.
If impotence occurs, it generally does not become an issue immediately.	An increased risk of developing rectal cancer.	
Good outcomes for early-stage cancer.		

Cryotherapy

Advantages	Disadvantages	Ideal candidate
Less invasive than surgery — no incision and minimal pain.	It is still considered experimental.	Men with early-stage cancer who do not have an active sex life, do not qualify for radiation therapy, and desire a minimally invasive alternative to surgery.
Quick recovery.	Risk of impotence is close to 100%.	
You can try another procedure if this one does not work.	Men with large prostates would have to undergo hormone therapy to shrink the prostate prior in order to have the procedure.	
Low risk of long-term incontinence.	Cure rates are lower than with other therapies.	

High-Intensity Focused Ultrasound

Advantages	Disadvantages	Ideal candidate
Has a high rate of preserving sexual function.	Still considered experimental in the United States.	Men with early- or intermediate-stage disease that is confined to the prostate.
If it doesn't work, other options are still open.	Little data exists on its long-term effectiveness.	
	Can involve urinary retention, a serious condition considered a medical emergency.	

Radical prostatectomy

Advantages	Disadvantages	Ideal candidate
Recurrence rates are lower than with any other therapy except brachytherapy.	Impotence without the loss of sexual interest. Drugs for erectile dysfunction can help in some cases.	A man with intermediate- or high-risk disease and a life expectancy of more than 10 years who already has problems with erectile dysfunction or has no strong interest in having an unimpaired sex life after surgery.
Easy to find a surgeon willing to remove the prostate gland.	Incontinence generally for a few weeks up to a year after surgery. Some permanent incontinence. Most men continue to have stress incontinence.	
	A long recovery of at least one month.	

Comparing your options *continued*

Nerve-sparing prostatectomy

Advantages	Disadvantages	Ideal candidate
The possibility, but not the assurance, of recovering full sexual function within a few months up to five years of surgery. If no cancer is thought to be left behind, the procedure is considered a surgical cure, although the risk of recurrence still exists.	All the risks that go with having a radical prostatectomy.	A younger, otherwise healthy man with high-risk disease and a desire to hopefully maintain sexual function after surgery.

Robotic prostatectomy

Advantages	Disadvantages	Ideal candidate
The same as for laparoscopic surgery, except the robotic method is considered more high-tech, with superior outcomes that are probably equal to or better than manual radical prostatectomy.	The long-term benefits and side effects are still unproven.	Same as for radical prostatectomy.

Laparoscopic prostatectomy

Advantages	Disadvantages	Ideal candidate
Faster recovery rate, less blood loss compared to manual radical surgery.	Generally inferior cure rates compared to radical prostatectomy.	Same as for radical prostatectomy.
Faster recovery of continence and, in nerve-sparing surgery, faster recovery of sexual function, compared to manual radical surgery.	The surgery is lengthy, meaning spending a longer amount of time under anesthesia.	
	If difficulties develop during the procedure, the surgeon may have to revert to a manual radical prostatectomy.	

Watchful waiting (for advanced disease)

Advantages	Disadvantages	Ideal candidate
Lack of treatment means little if any disruption in quality of life.	Treatment is limited to alleviating symptoms but not curing the disease.	Older men with advanced disease or men who are otherwise in poor health.

Assuring the best treatment for *you*: how to work with your doctor

6

Men make lousy patients.

This is *not* just a casual observation. When it comes to visiting the doctor, men tend to be too passive. Compared to women, studies reveal, men ask fewer questions and tend to offer less information about themselves and their health.

Researchers at the New England Medical Center in Boston demonstrated this not too long ago when they observed the behavior of 115 men and 181 women during a typical 15-minute visit to their primary care physician. They found that men asked their doctor only one question compared to women who asked an average of six questions.

This definitely is *not* the way you want to behave in front of the doctor checking out your prostate. Keeping your mouth shut is the last thing you want to do.

Here's why.

The most inconvenient truth

In most cases, diagnosing a prostate problem is relatively easy. The situation, however, starts to get touchy when you get to the bottom line: Determining the best treatment option for *you*.

As you now know, there is a mind-numbing array of options and treatments that address prostate troubles, ranging from active surveillance to drug therapy to surgery. Unfortunately, there is no one option that is decidedly the best and specialists don't agree on what is most effective. Also, as you've surely noticed, nearly all of them carry the risk of side effects, most notably impotence and incontinence.

> There is a bias against active surveillance because it carries a risk of a malpractice claim if the cancer should become aggressive, despite following medical guidelines.

Then there is this unfortunate reality: The treatment your doctor recommends may not necessarily be the best solution for you. There is well-documented evidence that your doctor just may recommend the treatment that is best for him — meaning the procedure that is standard or the procedure he is professionally trained to perform.

Just how widespread this "practice" is surfaced in 2010 when researchers in New Jersey analyzed the types of therapies used to treat 85,088 Medicare patients between the ages of 65 and 74 who had been diagnosed with prostate cancer.

"The type of treatment was strongly associated with the type of specialist consulted," says Thomas L. Jang, M.D., assistant professor of surgery at The Cancer Institute of New Jersey and the lead researcher in the study. The most frequent treatment performed on the more than 42,000 men who were seen by a urologist was a radical prostatectomy, the most aggressive and life-altering option. Radiation therapy was the most common treatment used on the men who saw both a radiation oncologist and a urologist.

Interestingly, the researchers noted that active surveillance — essentially doing nothing but monitor the disease with frequent checkups — turned out to be the treatment of choice only among the 20 percent who were also seeing their primary care physician during the time from diagnosis to treatment. Primary care physicians can play a role in helping guide the treatment decision.

This was the largest, but not the first, study to report on this type of physician behavior. A study published in the *Journal of the American Medical Association* more than 10 years ago asked 1,000 specialists what treatment they would recommend for a man with early-stage prostate cancer and a life expectancy of at least another 10 years. A total of 93 percent of urologists who specialize in surgery recommended surgery as the preferred treatment and 72 percent of radiation oncologists said radiation therapy and surgery were equally effective.

"Our findings provide new insight into the relationship between physician visit patterns and receipt of therapy," said Jang and his colleagues in the Medicare study, which was published in *Archives of Internal Medicine*. "The known preferences of prostate cancer specialists for the treatment they themselves deliver underscores the need to ensure that all men are well-informed and have access to balanced information prior to making this important treatment decision."

So what does all this mean to you?

Well, for starters, it means that you cannot be passive about your care. It means working with your doctor so he can make the right diagnosis and recommend the best treatment. It means asking your doctor about *all* your treatment options, and questioning his recommendation. And, no matter how much you trust your doctor, it means you should get a second opinion — and possibly a third or even a fourth, if necessary.

It also means making an appointment with your doctor as soon as you detect a problem and being proactive in your care right from the get-go.

Realize that the specialty of the physician who renders an opinion will bias his recommendation. If you meet the criteria for active surveillance, your primary care physician may be your best ally for following that protocol — not a urologist who performs many prostatectomies.

If major surgery or therapy is needed, brachytherapy may be the best option. But brachytherapy may not even be considered as an option unless a physician or group specializing in brachytherapy is consulted. Therefore, you may have to bring this to the attention of your doctor.

Finding a specialist

There are no hard and fast rules when it comes to picking a prostate specialist, but whom you see is important because it can impact how your problem will eventually be treated.

The most obvious place to start is by asking your primary care physician for a referral. Also, there are several sources on the Internet where you can check out a physician's background and history, including patient feedback, though some of these services charge a fee. To get started, just Google the name of the doctor who was recommended to you.

Make sure whomever you choose is included in your insurance plan and get it verified when you call for your appointment.

Help your urologist help you

Unless a prostate problem is detected during a routine exam or through a suspicious PSA reading, the most common reason a man ends up in a urologist's office is due to a change in his response to nature's call.

When you see your doctor, he'll want to know exactly what's been troubling you. You'll be helping him help you by showing up for your office visit fully prepared — not just with the questions you want to ask but with information that will help your doctor make an accurate diagnosis. That means being prepared with the most dependable and detailed information possible.

There is an advantage in this for you, as well. It's easy to get rattled and rushed in a doctor's office. Even the most important questions and obvious facts can disappear in the vacuum of a mind trying to wrap itself around the thought that life as you love it might change. So take some cool and collected time several days before your doctor's appointment to prepare the following.

A two- or three-day urination diary. Note the times of day you urinated, estimate how much you urinated, and what and how much you drank between trips to the bathroom. Report if you've had urinary leakage and what you were doing at the time it occurred. Also, note how pressing the urge was to urinate.

A list of symptoms. Check the list of symptoms associated with a prostate problem in the box *Symptoms of a sick prostate* on page 37 and make a record of all those you are experiencing or have experienced recently. Give as much detail as possible.

Your medical history. This is helpful if you're seeing this doctor for the first time or haven't seen this doctor in a long time. It's not necessary for you to collect medical records from every doctor you've seen. However, be prepared to furnish the following information:

- current medical conditions

- past illnesses, injuries, surgeries, and hospitalizations

- your history of catheterizations, if any

- medications — prescription and over-the-counter — that you are taking, including their dosages

- nutritional supplements you are taking, including their dosages

- allergies to foods or medicines that you may have

■ your history of taking over-the-counter cold and allergy medications

Summary of your recent sexual activity. Include the number of sexual partners you have or have had, the types of intercourse you engage in, and what kind of birth control, if any, you use. Most importantly, note if your typical sexual patterns have changed recently.

Too many tests

Are doctors overusing medical diagnostic testing tools?

Consider this: An estimated 10 billion laboratory tests and 500 million imaging procedures are performed in the United States each year. That comes to about 35 lab tests and two imaging exams per person.

Source: The Medical Mentor

Just routine procedure — or is it?

Depending on your symptoms and what your doctor learns from talking to you and reviewing your records, he will want to give you a physical and most likely order some tests, including a PSA test, before coming up with a diagnosis. For certain, you won't be leaving the office without getting a physical that includes a digital rectal exam. The doctor may even ask you to urinate so he can observe if the stream is strong, weak, or irregular.

During a physical exam, the doctor will press your lower abdomen to check for a possible mass. The digital rectal exam allows him to feel your prostate. The procedure, which takes less than a minute, involves inserting a lubricated gloved finger an inch or so into the rectum to feel the gland and assess its size and shape. If your doctor feels hardness on certain areas of the prostate, it raises the suspicion of cancer. If the prostate is soft and spongy, it's likely an infection, especially if you wince in pain. If it's enlarged, he can feel that as well. The doctor may suspect that your problem is not specifically your prostate, but rather an infection involving your urinary system, bladder, or kidneys. Only certain tests will confirm his suspicions.

The operative word here is *certain*. In most instances you will not need more than a test or two to figure out what is wrong with you. For example, a simple urinalysis can confirm benign prostatic hyperplasia in men with mild symptoms. If your doctor recommends a battery of tests, ask how they will benefit your diagnosis. Why? Because there is ample evidence indicating doctors are overusing diagnostic testing, especially imaging tests that expose you to radiation.

While the average American typically is not exposed to too much radiation, the National Council on Radiation Protection and Measurements (NCRP) has found that we are now being exposed to more than seven times as much ionizing radiation from medical procedures than we were in the early 1980s. This is of enough concern that the NCRP has officially cautioned doctors to weigh the merits of exposure before proceeding with a test.

"The rising number of malpractice lawsuits has created a climate in which physicians are motivated both by their desire to get the best treatment for their patients and by the perceived need to have a paper trail proving that no stone was left unturned," says Bob Sheff, M.D., a patient advocate and author of *The Medical Mentor: Get the Health Care You Deserve in Today's Medical System*. "Rather than just do the test they feel is most appropriate, many physicians are practicing 'defensive medicine,' and doing tests that they believe are only remotely useful."

So you may be wondering, what's wrong with extra testing that doesn't expose you to radiation but offers you double or triple assurance of a correct diagnosis — especially if your insurance will pay for it?

For one, diagnostic testing, just like treatment, carries risk. Also, it increases the risk of conflicting results, which could lead to more tests. Most likely, in the end, your doctor will default to the test considered "standard procedure."

Also, diagnostic testing is expensive and makes a major contribution to the escalating cost of health care in the United States.

For every test ordered there should be a direct benefit to your health. "A test is only necessary if it will aid in your care," says Dr. Sheff. "You need to know how the information will affect your diagnosis and treatment."

Dr. Sheff recommends asking your doctors these questions when a test is ordered:

- What impact will this test have on the management of my care?

- What are the benefits and risk of the test?

- Is this the proper time in the management of my care to have this test?

- Is this test covered by my medical insurance?

If your doctor doesn't know the answer to the last question for sure, check with your insurance carrier before agreeing to the test.

But he's just a kid!

Question: Is it better to pick a doctor who is young, full of enthusiasm, and up on the latest techniques, or an older doctor with years of experience?

Answer: The best physician will usually be one who is neither too young nor too old. You want a physician who is caring, intelligent, well-trained, and stays current in his field, says patient advocate Bob Sheff, M.D., author of *The Medical Mentor.*

Why you want a second opinion

You could say that medicine is both an art and a science. Science, you see, is based on objectivity — that is, reaching a conclusion without prejudgment. Art is subjective. Medicine is a little bit of both — and nowhere is it more muddled than when it comes to treating prostate problems, and prostate cancer in particular. "Selecting the appropriate treatment can be challenging, since no therapy has emerged as clearly superior," says Dr. Jang, assistant professor of surgery at The Cancer Institute of New Jersey.

Treatment — the science — is based on the art of interpreting the results of diagnostic tests. And opinions clash, even at the world's best prostate treatment centers. A case in point is a study conducted at Johns Hopkins University Medical Center that involved the pathology reports of 535 men scheduled to have a radical prostatectomy.

Johns Hopkins independently had its own pathologists review the reports and found that seven of the biopsies were misclassified. Further study revealed that six out of the seven weren't even cancer and the surgeries were called off. (For the record, the purpose of the study was to find out if reviewing biopsies would save the cost of unnecessary surgery, not to monitor the skill of pathologists.)

An accurate pathology reading is essential because it is the basis for treatment decisions. Spotting cancerous prostate cells and determining how abnormal they appear can be difficult.

Findings, such as the Johns Hopkins' study, and the reality of human error are why it is important to get a second opinion when the diagnosis is prostate cancer or prostate surgery.

Don't hesitate to tell the doctor making your diagnosis that you would like a second opinion. He may, in fact, bring it up before you ask. Most doctors today are open to patients seeking a second opinion. Most insurers will pay, but make sure to check with your insurance company.

You can ask for a referral from the doctor who made your diagnosis or from your primary care physician. Make sure to keep your primary care doctor involved in the decision-making process. As with the men in the Medicare study, it could make the difference between active surveillance and invasive surgery.

If it's possible (and it should be), ask for a referral to a doctor who is not affiliated with the same hospital or practice, as doctors within the same institution tend to share similar points of view. Also, ask to see someone whose expertise is in a different therapy. For example, if you've been diagnosed with prostate cancer by a urologist who recommends a prostatectomy, see an oncologist whose expertise is in a possibly superior therapy such as brachytherapy, radiation seed therapy.

To make the process go smoothly, make arrangements to have your file and diagnostic records sent to your second opinion doctor prior to your appointment. Your doctor can either give them to you to take with you to your appointment or send them directly to the doctor.

During the consultation, the doctor will review the information with you and perform another physical. He may even want to order some more tests. A report with his evaluation will be shared with you and the referring physician.

The buddy system is best

Four ears are better than two when it comes to listening to what your doctor has to say — especially when you are facing the likelihood of cancer or surgery. Ask your spouse or a good friend to go with you to the appointment. This person will be your second set of ears. He or she can also take notes.

Afterwards, compare notes and impressions while they are still fresh in your minds.

Find out about all your options

Ask your doctors — this includes your referral doctor, second-opinion doctor, and your primary care physician — to tell you about all the treatment options and their advantages and disadvantages, including risks and side effects. If the doctors don't agree on what is the best treatment for you, or if you suspect your doctor is biased toward his own treatment specialty, try this approach.

- Ask the doctors to explain to you why and how they came to their respective conclusions.

- Request that the specialists discuss your diagnosis with each other and try to come to an acceptable consensus.

- If a consensus is not reached, ask your primary care physician or enlist the help of a third specialist to help you sort through your options.

- Consider seeking an opinion at a nationally recognized treatment center such as those listed in Part 4 of this book or one affiliated with the National Comprehensive Cancer Network at *www.nccn.org*.

15 questions to ask a surgeon

When a doctor recommends surgery, there are two questions that you should get answered right away.

1. Do I really *need* surgery? And,

2. Do I really need *this* surgery?

If the answer to both is yes, it is in your best interest to continue with these questions.

3. Why do I need this surgery?

4. What are the alternatives to this surgery?

5. What will it mean to my prognosis if I don't have the surgery you are recommending?

6. What are the risks of the procedure you're recommending?

7. How many surgeries of this type have you done?

8. What is your success rate?

9. How are you defining your success rate?

10. Does the surgery require hospitalization?

11. What are the side effects of the surgery?

12. Will I need to be catheterized after surgery and, if so, for how long?

13. How long will I be incapacitated?

14. How will the surgery affect my sex life?

15. Will I become incontinent?

Finally, don't feel rushed into making a decision. Unless it's a medical emergency, meaning you need treatment *now!*, you have time to study and consider your options. Even with prostate cancer, time is generally on your side because the cancer grows slowly. In the end, the decision is yours — and you are the one who will have to live with the results.

Quality of life issue: getting help for incontinence

Incontinence isn't life-threatening, but it is life-altering. For many men it is devastating. It can have such a profound effect on men who undergo prostate surgery that it leaves many of them depressed and socially withdrawn.

Urinary *difficulties* are common to all prostate disease. They represent the package of symptoms for benign prostatic hyperplasia (BPH), but *true incontinence* — that is, the inability to maintain urinary control — is a rare complication only in men with severe BPH, and it is almost never heard of as a complication of prostatitis. However, incontinence is a high-risk consequence of surgery for prostate cancer. Incontinence that lingers for more than a year is considered permanent.

Though most men will experience some urinary difficulties immediately following surgery, studies show the rates of incontinence after one year for various treatments are:

■ robotic surgery: 10%

■ radical and nerve-sparing prostatectomy: 8%

- cryotherapy: 5%

- brachytherapy (radioactive seeds): less than 1%

- external beam radiation therapy: less than 1%

These near-zero statistics for men undergoing radiation therapy, unfortunately, don't mean there is no risk of urinary difficulties. Radiation and radioactive seeds have a small risk of burning the urethra and causing urethritis, a condition similar to a urinary tract infection that carries its own set of problems. There is also a risk that radioactive seeds will damage the urethra, but it won't be noticed until the cumulative effects of the radiation take hold. If scarring results, then the muscles can lose some of their ability to control urine flow. With cryotherapy there is a risk that part of the urethra or nearby bladder will be frozen and damaged by the procedure.

Although rare these days, radiation also carries the risk of burning the rectum, resulting in chronic proctitis, a rectal condition characterized by painful and loose bowel movements. It can lead to fecal incontinence. As you can imagine, this can cause an even greater strain on quality of life.

Why incontinence is a risk

The prostate and the urethra are like Siamese twins. They are stuck together for life, or at least that is the way nature intended it to be. The urethra, the vessel that carries urine from the bladder and out of the body, passes right through the prostate. You can live without your prostate (though some men will argue this), but you can't live without expelling urine from your body. So prostate surgery means the two must be separated — a delicate procedure that requires practiced guidance in such a compact space. There isn't much room for error. Studies show the degree of incontinence following surgery has a lot to do with the skill of the surgeon.

Once the prostate is removed, the surgeon must then reattach the urethra to the bladder. A little piece of the prostate near the bladder wall must be left intact to help secure the urethra. If there are undetected cancer cells in the area, then cancer will be left behind. Depending on the size of the tumor or the anatomy of the prostate, the surgeon might have to remove some tissue at the adjoining bladder neck, a ring of muscles that prevent urine from leaking out of the bladder. These muscles affect how well the new connection between the bladder and the urethra come together.

If a tumor is large, it may also mean removing a part of the sphincter, the muscle that works like a hatch to stop and start urine flow. Surgery sometimes can damage the nerves that control the sphincter. The extent to which the prostate cancer involves the sphincter is a major factor that will determine whether or not you will have urinary problems.

After surgery, a catheter is placed in the urethra for a few days. This in itself will cause temporary urinary difficulties. A catheter raises the risk of urinary tract infection and urinary retention.

4 kinds of incontinence

Incontinence is classified as four conditions and they are all involved in prostate disease.

Stress incontinence. If you laugh, sneeze, cough, or bend over and, *whoops*, a little urine seeps into your underwear, you have stress incontinence. It's a common problem that sneaks up on you as you get older and it is a fact of life for a lot of men who have had prostate surgery. Stress incontinence is caused by a weakness in the sphincter muscle that opens and shuts to control urine flow.

Urge incontinence. You feel the need to urinate and the urge suddenly gets so bad you can barely make it to the bathroom in time. Sometimes you don't. This is urge incontinence.

Overflow incontinence. You have to go but you really can't, then the bladder gets so full, you unexpectedly start to drip, drip, drip. Overflow incontinence occurs when you are unable to completely empty your bladder and it is a common problem associated with BPH. The leakage can cause you discomfort and even embarrassment, but this isn't nearly as troublesome as the potential problems it can create. Urine left in the bladder is a breeding ground for bacteria that can cause infection. If ignored, the problem can also damage the bladder.

Mixed incontinence. This is a combination of stress and urge incontinence and is among the classic symptoms of BPH and a common side effect of surgical removal of the prostate.

Symptoms of urethritis

Urethritis is an infection of the urethra that is generally picked up through sexual contact, but it can also occur as a complication of brachytherapy. Its symptoms are similar to prostatitis, but more severe.

- watery discharge from penis
- a "glued shut" appearance at the opening of the penis
- discharge from the penis that leaves a brownish or yellowish stain on the front of the underwear
- an itchy feeling inside the penis
- discomfort in the penis during urination

The condition is treated with antibiotics. You can also use the same self-help ideas as for prostatitis. You can find them on page 77.

Surgery and incontinence

Incontinence after surgery is usually the result of one of the following complications.

Bladder spasms. Surgery can cause a buildup of high pressure in the bladder as it fills, creating spasms that cause urge incontinence, frequent urination, and nighttime accidents. This is the most common complication of surgery. Half of all men with incontinence after surgery get bladder spasms.

Damage to the sphincter muscle. When the sphincter is damaged during surgery it can cause stress incontinence. This is a problem in 35 percent of men with post-surgical incontinence.

A combination of bladder malfunction and sphincter damage. This results in mixed incontinence and occurs in 10 percent of men who undergo surgery.

No matter how you're feeling, try as hard as you can to not let incontinence get you down. It's not the end of the world, or more precisely, *your* world. In most cases, your incontinence problems will resolve on their own, and even if they don't, there are treatments that work adequately enough that you can carry on with your life without fear of an accident or embarrassment.

No single treatment works for everyone. Your treatment options for incontinence will depend on the type and severity of your problem. When considering your options, you should take your lifestyle into account. Almost always, your doctor will urge you to start with simple treatment options. Many men have found that they can regain urinary control by changing a few habits and doing exercises to strengthen the muscles that hold urine in the bladder. If behavioral techniques do not work, you might be a candidate for medication or a continence device that is implanted surgically. Despite potential problems, surgery may be the best choice in certain circumstances.

Start with small artillery

Before you go to drastic measures, doctors recommend that you first try managing the problem on your own. Simple changes in your lifestyle can help control your problem and maintain a respectable quality of life. A recent study in the *Journal of the American Medical Association* found that behavioral strategies reduced the number of incontinence episodes by 50 percent in men who had undergone prostate surgery. You can give some or all of these time-tested remedies a try.

Depend on a hidden helper. Wearing absorbent pads or adult diapers should not be an embarrassment. Think of them as security to save yourself from embarrassment until the techniques you are working on start to take hold. There are many different products on the market including pads, shields, guards, and bladder-control briefs. They are relatively inexpensive and can be purchased at your local pharmacy. Try different brands until you find a product that best meets your needs.

When wearing this kind of protection, you need to take special care of your skin, as wet urine against the skin can cause irritation or a rash that could become infected. To avoid this problem, do the following.

- Remove wet articles as soon as possible.

- Cleanse the skin with soap and warm water.

- Rinse well and pat dry.

- Apply a protective cream or ointment to prevent dryness.

Down with the alcohol and caffeine. Down the drain, that is. Doctors will tell you these are the first things to give up. Both are diuretics, which means they increase the amount of urine your body produces. They can also irritate the bladder.

Out with acidic and spicy foods. Acidic foods such as grapefruit and tomatoes, as well as a lot of spices, are also irritating to the bladder. If you notice that these foods are creating more urinary urgency, cut them out of your diet.

Learn the benefits of bladder training. If you are undergoing surgery, the sooner you start using these techniques, the better your chances of making your urinary problems short-term. Bladder training offers big benefits. You can learn to control your urge to urinate, lengthen the amount of time between bathroom trips, and increase the amount of urine your bladder can hold. Studies found it decreased urge incontinence in men by an average of 75 percent.

The following techniques are proven to be effective, but you must have patience. It can take one to three months before you notice the difference. You might want to keep a diary of your bathroom trips, mistakes and all, so your doctor can help guide you and assess your progress.

Scheduled urination teaches you to go to the bathroom at specific times throughout the day. Start by forcing yourself to urinate every half hour, whether you have the urge or not. Gradually increase the time by five or 10 minutes until you can go at least two or three hours without an accident. Depending on your control, you may be able to eventually go longer.

Delayed urination can help men with urge incontinence show the sphincter who's boss. The technique can be a little tricky at first. Start by trying to hold your urine for five minutes when you feel a need to go to the bathroom. When five minutes gets easy, increase the waiting time to 10 minutes. Do this until your hold time is three to four hours between bathroom visits.

To help control the urge while in your holding pattern, shut your eyes and concentrate on your breathing. Take slow deep breaths.

Relax your way to urinary control. If you have urge incontinence and are constantly racing for the bathroom, this tactic will help you build physical and mental control.

- Stop.

- Relax your stomach muscles.

- Concentrate on waiting.

- Once the urge has passed, walk, don't run, to the bathroom.

Exercise your pelvis and penis. These Kegel exercises are particularly helpful for getting back urinary control after a radical prostatectomy. They should be started as soon as possible after surgery.

You start by identifying the two sets of muscles you will be working. One group is located around the rectum but is used to stop the flow of urine. The other group is at the base of the penis. These are the muscles you usually contract when you are trying to get the last few drips out after a trip to the bathroom. To do the exercises properly, you contract the muscles near your rectum first, hold them tight, and then contract the penis muscles. It might take some practice and concentration, but you'll get the hang of it. Here's how to go about the exercises.

- First thing in the morning, urinate in only very small amounts, contracting the muscles in your pelvis every few seconds, at least five times, to stop the stream. Do this until your bladder is empty.

- Throughout the day, practice contracting and releasing these muscles even when you're not urinating. Hold them tight for about 10 seconds, relax, and repeat about 15 times. Do this six times a day.

- Practice every time you urinate until you can do it easily.

- Whenever you are in a situation that normally causes leakage, such as lifting or coughing, consciously tighten these muscles.

Beat incontinence with biofeedback. If you're having trouble getting the hang of Kegel exercises, ask your doctor about biofeedback. Even if you've mastered Kegels, biofeedback can increase the effectiveness of the exercises.

Biofeedback teaches you how to instinctively recognize involuntary changes in your body, such as the need to urinate, and use your mind to control them. It's a high-tech version of bladder training and it requires special instrumentation and a trained behavioral specialist to teach you.

For about six weeks you'll undergo half-hour training sessions wearing a special undergarment with sensing electrodes that will help you isolate the right muscles involved in urination and improve their strength. Biofeedback has been found to help immensely in regaining urinary control.

Your doctor can guide you to a biofeedback specialist in your vicinity.

Visualize yourself with continence. We all use our imagination from time to time to get us out of a jam. By using a special imaging technique called visualization, you may be able to mentally see your way back to a continent life.

Visualization has been used for hundreds of years by alternative healers as a means to soothe, calm, heal, and control the body. It involves capturing a mental image of the state you want to achieve and concentrating on it in the absence of all other images and thoughts.

Practitioners of visualization believe the power of concentration can transfer to real life. For example, if you have urge incontinence you might picture a dam holding back a river. The emergency need to go to the bathroom will eventually subside. If you have overflow incontinence and visualize turning off a faucet tighter and tighter, you'll eventually learn how to squeeze back annoying dribbles.

Many people can learn the technique easily on their own, but others need the guidance of a book, a learning center, or a psychotherapist.

Bringing out the brigade

Incontinence doesn't have to be a fact of life for the rest of your life. If natural techniques don't help, your doctor will do some testing to get to the source and severity of your problems. Depending on the outcome of the tests, you could be offered any one of these options. Keep in mind, some of these options, especially surgery, have serious risks.

Medication. Medications can help control mild to moderate incontinence but drugs have not been found to be effective for severe cases. If your incontinence is caused by bladder spasms and the urethra is not damaged, medication could be your solution. A class of prescription drugs called anticholinergics can help relax the bladder and eliminate spasms. They include oxybutynin (Ditropan and the Oxytrol patch) and tolterodine tartrate (Detrol).

Nasal decongestants, such as pseudoephedrine (Chlor Trimeton) and the antidepressant imipramine (Tofranil) can help reduce stress incontinence by strengthening bladder neck muscles.

Collagen injections. Collagen injections are popular in the cosmetic industry as a way of expanding facial skin to smooth out fine lines. It works in a similar fashion in urology by bulking up the muscles around the bladder neck to prevent urinary leakage.

The process involves getting two or three injections initially and repeating them every four months to a year, depending on how effective the treatments are. They are usually administered using local anesthesia.

Collagen is the substance that gives skin its elasticity. The collagen used for injections is taken from cattle.

Penile clamps. This do-it-yourself device keeps the shaft of the penis shut so that urine cannot accidentally escape. All you do is insert the device halfway down the shaft of the penis and then tighten it to compress the urethra. You remove it about every two hours to go to the bathroom and you don't wear it at all while sleeping.

It is not as bizarre or painful as it may sound. However, there are some downsides. If it is left on too long, it can cause strictures, a type of scarring with its own set of complications. If clamped too tight it can cut off blood circulation. You'll also need to examine your penis frequently to make sure the clamp is not causing any injury or infection. If it's causing a problem, you'll know it. Pain, itching, discharge, and trouble emptying your bladder are the symptoms.

Bladder pacemaker. You've heard of a pacemaker for the heart, well, this works in a similar fashion. It uses a tiny device to electrically control the nerve impulses in the bladder that turn on and off the spigot. It is used to control urge incontinence.

Installing the device is a two-stage process. In the first stage, the surgeon implants a tiny electrode next to the main nerve that controls the bladder and attaches it to a pacemaker that you'll wear on your belt for the next week or so. The pacemaker sends mild electrical pulses to the nerve to help control an erratic bladder. Once it gets in its pace, a second procedure is done in which a pacemaker is programmed and implanted under the skin, usually in the buttocks. A hand-held electromagnetic device activates the nerve stimulator and can be adjusted to strengthen the signal.

The bladder pacemaker, which is implanted on an outpatient basis, is estimated to work in about 80 percent of people who try it. The procedure can be reversed without any effect on the nerve.

Artificial urinary sphincter. Yes, this is exactly what it sounds like — a prosthetic sphincter — and it is generally reserved as the procedure to use when all else fails. The prosthesis consists of three parts: an elongated cuff that fits around and substitutes for the damaged urethra, a pressure-regulating balloon that is placed in the abdomen to maintain pressure on the cuff, and a pump that is placed in the scrotum so that the cuff can be deflated and open the sphincter so you can urinate. Tubes connect the three parts.

The cuff remains inflated until you have to go to the bathroom. When its time to go, you squeeze the device in the scrotum to activate the pump, which deflates the cuff, sending fluid from the bladder and out the hatch. The cuff automatically reinflates in 30 seconds.

The artificial sphincter has been around for about 20 years and is shown to have about an 85 percent satisfaction rate.

Male sling. A newer, less invasive procedure for men with sphincter damage is the male sling, a device that compresses the urethra to keep urine from leaking uncontrollably.

In this procedure, the surgeon makes an incision in the perineum, the space between the scrotum and rectum, and implants three titanium bone screws on either side of the pubic bone. The surgeon attaches a suture to each screw and weaves a sling-like device that acts like a closure for the urethra.

The sling is not a compressor but rather a supportive device that lifts the urethra and allows the sphincter to work more efficiently. The additional support prevents the abdominal pressure that causes urine to escape when you laugh, cough, or bend over.

Because the device is so new, there is not a lot of data on its effectiveness, but according to the Prostate Cancer Research Institute, "results with the male sling have been encouraging." In one study, 40 percent of men using the sling reported complete dryness and 40 percent reported significant improvement. The other 20 percent were considered failures.

A word on proctitis

If radiation damages the rectum it can cause chronic proctitis, a painful inflammation of the rectum that leaves you with the constant feeling that you need to release your bowels. It can also lead to fecal incontinence. The symptoms include:

- rectal bleeding

- rectal pain

- pain when passing your bowels

- mucus in bowel movements

- diarrhea

- pain in the left side of the stomach

- a feeling of fullness in the rectum

Mild cases of proctitis caused by radiation burn generally will resolve on their own and don't require treatment. However, this is not a call you should make on your own, so see your doctor.

Conditions that include bleeding are usually treated with the steroid drug hydrocortisone and prescription anti-inflammatory medications, such as mesalamine (Apriso), sulfasalazine (Azulfidine), and olsalazine (Dipentum). In some cases, laser surgery may be recommended to burn away lesions.

Rekindling your love life: a sex survival guide

Let's be honest. When most men hear the words prostate cancer, the thought of death might flash through their heads, but what they also fear — what strikes terror in the loins and keeps them awake at night — is impotence. To some guys, impotence is a fate worse than death.

Study after study affirms that a man's ability to perform sexually defines his persona — his self-esteem, his self-confidence, his demeanor, his happiness. When he can't perform, they can all go down the tubes.

Impotence, or erectile dysfunction as doctors and television commercials call it these days, is defined as consistent failure to experience sexual intercourse due to the inability to have an erection hard enough to penetrate the vagina. Though an enlarged prostate or an infection can sometimes make this difficult and even painful, they do not necessarily cause permanent impotence. The treatments for prostate diseases frequently do cause temporary or permanent impotence — and the most notorious is radical surgery for prostate cancer. Impotence doesn't occur in all men all the time, at least not permanently, but it is much more common than a lot of surgeons like to admit.

While treatment can take your ability to have an erection, it doesn't take away your desire to make love. Androgen deprivation therapy, used for prostate cancer, is the only treatment that zaps your libido, and it is generally only used in advanced cases when other treatments fail. So you can see why the fear of impotence is so entwined in a man's decision on what treatment to choose for an ailing prostate and why it creates so much anguish when the fear becomes reality.

The mechanics of an erection set

An erection is a highly orchestrated mind-body event with all the suspense of a one-act play. Though many an off-color joke has been made about a man thinking with his penis, in a way it really isn't all that far from the truth. Contrary to popular humor, however, it's the big brain that tells the little brain what to do.

An erection begins in the conscious brain when erotic stimulation, either real or imagined, sends impulses down the central nervous system that tell the nerve bundles sitting on the outer edge of the prostate gland to let the fun begin. Just like a hydraulic system that raises the curtain on a Broadway stage, these nerves release a chemical called cyclic guanosine monophosphate (cGMP) that forces blood vessels in the penis to open the floodgates. On cue, blood flows into two chambers that run the length of the penis called the corpora cavernosa, making the organ get longer, wider, and harder, then stiff and erect. It's showtime. As long as the blood stays in the chambers, the performance goes on. When you have an orgasm, another chemical called phosphodiesterase type 5 (PDE5) breaks down cGMP and makes the erection subside. The show's over.

These chemicals, nerve bundles, and blood vessels play leading roles in making and sustaining an erection. If the blood vessels or nerves are compromised or damaged in any way, blood flow is impeded. The show can't go on. Without nerves, there is no electricity to spark the chemistry. Either way, it's curtains for your love life. You've got erectile dysfunction.

From trauma to traumatic

It doesn't take a doctor to diagnose impotence. When you're aroused and nothing rises time and time again, the problem is obvious. You're among the millions of unlucky guys whose prostate treatment has robbed them of their masculinity, or has made the once-spontaneous pleasure of making love an anxiety-ridden, arduous task.

Any prostate treatment, even a minimally invasive procedure, is traumatic and can carry residual side effects that affect your ability to have an erection. They can take time to resolve, or may never be resolved completely. Doctors admit that even the most expertly performed nerve-sparing radical prostatectomy can cause injury to the nerve bundles. For example, tiny, delicate nerves can get injured when the surgeon stretches them back and out of the way to remove the prostate. Or a surgeon can inadvertently cause an injury when trying to control the high degree of bleeding that is common in prostate surgery. Sometimes, the heat used to cauterize and reconnect the urethra can burn nerve fibers.

Any of these things can harm nerve fibers and cause a loss of sensitivity that weakens the electrical impulses that spark an erection. Over time, lack of adequate stimulation can cause the spongy tissue of the corpora cavernosa to deteriorate. Like an elastic waistband that never gets stretched, it loses its give. Erections get weaker and weaker or difficult to maintain.

Even when a prostate procedure is declared to be a success, and you no longer have a detectable PSA, the victory is more bitter than sweet if your love life exists only in your memory.

Compounding the problem is the humiliation and shame that make most men suffer in silence. For many men it causes psychological problems and shatters relationships. Impotence, however, is nothing to hide in a closest. It's a quite common problem, even among men who haven't been through a prostate ordeal. One study found that 50 percent of men in mid-life have some degree of erectile dysfunction and 90 percent of them don't admit it even to their doctor — a big mistake if you value your love life. Millions of men who have taken their problem to a doctor have found a solution that works to their sexual satisfaction.

Thanks to medical science, there is a way for just about every man to become sexually fulfilled again, no matter what the cause of his impotence. The longer you allow the problem to linger, however, the more troublesome it can be to overcome.

Erections and orgasm: what gives?

An erection and an orgasm are mutually exclusive. Just like you can have an erection and never reach orgasm, you can have an orgasm without getting an erection. If you have had your prostate, seminal vesicles, and the neurovascular nerves removed, it doesn't necessarily have an effect on your sex drive, the ability to have an orgasm, or the sensation of the climax. It only destroys your ability to have an erection. The other thing you'll notice is the absence of semen. Your orgasm will be dry. You will be infertile.

Consider your state of stress

Impotence that results from prostate treatment is a physical problem, but psychological factors can make an already troubling situation even worse.

Subconscious or even conscious fears about your prostate disease may interfere with your ability to perform. For example, some men with prostate cancer may avoid sex because they worry that tumor cells can be transplanted sexually. Or men with chronic bacterial prostatitis may worry about spreading an infection. Be assured that this is nothing to worry about. Cancer is unique to the individual. It cannot be spread sexually or otherwise to others. Though prostatitis rarely can be infectious, it is never contagious, unless it is a consequence of a sexually transmitted disease.

Some men who have successfully been treated for prostate cancer worry about having sex because they are concerned that increases in testosterone levels may cause the cancer to recur. Wrong again. Testosterone fuels your desire to make love, but having sex does not increase testosterone levels. If any of these fears interfere with your sexual performance, put them to bed permanently. They are nothing more than myths and misconceptions.

There are, however, issues — psychological, physical, and environmental — that can slow down men otherwise capable of having an erection; so imagine what they can do to someone who lacks all or some of the nerves or other necessary equipment. Consider these factors. If any of them apply to you, doing something about it might help improve your sexual stamina.

Rate your performance. Emotional stress plays a big role in your ability to perform sexually. Consider what's been going on in your life — how you're handling your illness, what's going on with your job, the effect your illness is having on your wife or significant other, your financial stability. Where do they all stand now in comparison to your way of life when your sex life was in high gear?

Slow down on the drinking. Though a single drink can help loosen inhibitions and maybe even help put you in the mood for love, too much alcohol has the opposite effect. It's well-known that as blood alcohol rises, it impairs judgment and sensory perception, and this includes the nervous system. Also, when drinking in moderation turns into excessive drinking, it can impair the function of the nerves that control an erection.

Put out the cigarettes. Nicotine decreases blood flow in the arteries and can interfere with the relaxation of smooth muscles that allow blood to flood the penis.

Recreational drugs stop the fun. Whatever high a recreational drug may deliver becomes disappointment in the bedroom. Studies show a link between impotence and drug addiction.

Don't let depression keep you down. Depression is common among men who've gone through a medical prostate ordeal and it is not just exclusive to men who've had cancer. Depression automatically dampens the romantic flame and most antidepressants also tend to depress libido. If you're depressed for whatever reason, or experiencing anxiety due to your illness, seeking counseling may help get you out of the doldrums.

Be good to your heart. Hardening of the arteries that puts you at an increased risk of heart attack and stroke can also affect the arteries in your southern hemisphere. If you have any degree of blockage in your heart or another vascular problem, it can also show up in your penis as an inability to get a strong erection. Over time, it can result in no erection at all.

Consider taking niacin (nicotinic acid). Time-release regular niacin may help blood flow not only through the coronary arteries, but also into other blood vessels involved in erections, according to anecdotal reports. It's even reported to be helpful in cases of Raynaud's disease when there is poor circulation in the hands.

The prescription drug Niaspan (extended-release niacin) is often prescribed to improve circulation in those at risk for heart disease. Slo-Niacin is an over-the-counter time-release niacin that has not been through the demanding FDA approval process, but, nevertheless, may have similar benefits. Don't be fooled by "flush-free" niacin (inositol hexaniacinate) or Nicomide (nicotinamide). They do not have the same beneficial effect on circulation as regular and time-release niacin.

Keep your sugar under control. Diabetes, a blood sugar problem caused by impaired insulin production, is an insidious and devastating disease because it threatens so many aspects of life. Over time it can damage the nerves and blood supply to the penis. Estimates show as many as 75 percent of men with diabetes have erection problems within 10 years of developing the disease.

Consider a past injury. Damage to the neurovascular bundles that trigger an erection are a certain inflation fighter, but any kind of injury or disorder involving the central nervous system can weaken nerve impulses that affect erections. This includes damage from poorly fitted bicycle seats to conditions such as Parkinson's disease and multiple sclerosis.

Watch your weight. Obesity makes you sluggish for a variety of reasons. Fat and the clogged arteries caused by eating too much fat can slow circulation. Obesity can interfere with blood flow to the penis, making erections weak.

Figure in medications you are taking. Medications for high blood pressure, heart disease, depression, and allergies are the most common of the more than 200 prescription drugs that can make getting an erection more difficult. The effect is cumulative if you're taking a combination of these drugs. Check with your doctor to find out if erectile dysfunction is a risk for any medications you are taking. If you suspect a prescription medication is contributing to your problem, do not stop taking it. Talk to your doctor to find a possible solution that does not put your health at risk.

Get real. Consider yourself fortunate if your love life gets back to where it was prior to treatment, even if you go through a long streak of "no can do." The best-case scenario, doctors say, is that your sex life, as you knew it before treatment, will return. Don't count on it getting better. Younger men have the best chance of making a full recovery.

ED and the aging myth

True, getting an erection can get more difficult as you age, but there is enough scientific evidence to convince researchers that erectile dysfunction (ED) is not necessarily a consequence of aging. Erection problems are caused by health problems associated with aging, such as heart disease, poor circulation, and nerve disorders. In fact, erection troubles can be a sign of an undetected life-threatening illness. So don't ignore erectile dysfunction. Discuss it with your doctor.

Back in the saddle again

If you're experiencing erection problems as a result of prostate treatment, swallow your pride and see a doctor as soon as possible. The urologist or surgeon who treated your prostate disease can offer you solutions or refer you to a specialist in sexual dysfunction. Because erectile dysfunction is now recognized as a medical condition, your primary care physician should also be knowledgeable about treatment options.

If you are having disappointment in the bedroom and have been treated for a prostate problem, even if it was years ago, the two are probably related. Some men don't connect their impotence to their prostate because it can sometimes take months or even years after treatment for problems to develop. This is especially true for some men who have elected radiation or seed implants as treatment for prostate cancer, though impotence from radiation burn is no longer common. Men who have undergone less invasive treatments for cancer or other prostate problems may find their erections are weak or are not entirely there. Men who have had their nerves or smooth muscles damaged face the greatest challenge, but there are options that work for them.

If you're going to investigate options that can restore your love life, keep these thoughts in mind.

Don't delay. The sooner you address the problem, the better your chances are of ending up with a satisfactory outcome. Studies show that men recover their sexuality faster if they address the problem right after they recover from surgery or treatment.

Don't give up. Be forewarned that what works for one man may not work for another. Also, what doesn't work now may very well work in a few weeks or few months. Using the therapy properly — and this includes drugs — can take practice.

Involve your mate. Include your significant other in your discussions and the decision-making process. Impotence is a couple's problem, and she may be feeling the adjustment just as you are.

Beware of aphrodisiacs. When there are herbs and other natural medications advertised to help improve blood circulation and increase your libido, they most likely will do little or nothing if your problems are damaged nerves and blood pressure issues. Consult your doctor before you waste your money. If it sounds too good to be true, it probably is.

Here are accepted treatment options for men with erectile dysfunction.

Oral medication: vitamin V for victory

When sildenafil, best known by its brand name Viagra, hit the market in 1998, it was an overwhelming financial success for the pharmaceutical business. Yearly sales, since the drug has been approved, have been many billions of dollars.

Sildenafil, which was followed by two other drugs, tadalafil (Cialis) and vardenafil (Levitra), can achieve what no other impotence aid has been able to do — enable a man to get an erection naturally, while allowing that without sexual stimulation, nothing happens. All you do is pop the pill in advance of your anticipated rendezvous and no one is the wiser. The only discomfort may be the $10 or so you paid for the pill — although priapism, a prolonged and painful erection, is occasionally a side effect.

These oral medications belong to a group of drugs called PDE5 inhibitors. PDE5 is the acronym for phosphodiesterase type 5, the enzyme that breaks down the chemical cyclic guanosine monophosphate (cGMP) that makes the smooth muscle in the penis relax so blood can enter and make an erection. The way PDE5 inhibitors work is simple. They boost the staying power of cGMP by inhibiting PDE5 from doing its job. As a result, erections are strong and have staying power.

Though PDE5 inhibitors are dependable and effective, they do not work for everyone. Unfortunately, men who have had their nerves removed during a radical prostatectomy will not respond to these drugs. Also, erections may be hard to achieve if nerves or blood vessels have been damaged or compromised in any way. Studies show that even men who have had nerve-sparing surgery may be slow to respond to these drugs, but most eventually should.

If you qualify for PDE5 therapy, your doctor will work with you to prescribe the right pill and appropriate dosage. Studies show that for some men, taking the pill every day just as you would a blood pressure medication is the best way to beat impotence.

PDE5 inhibitors are potent medicine. Keep these precautions in mind when taking the drug.

Viagra and BPH medicines don't mix. PDE5 inhibitors do not mix with some medications, including certain drugs for benign prostatic hyperplasia (BPH). For example, you can't take Levitra if you are taking an alpha blocker for BPH. You can take Viagra, but not within four hours of taking an alpha blocker. You can't take either Levitra or Cialis if you're taking tamsulosin (Flomax), but you can take low-dose Viagra.

Be cautious if you have heart disease. If you have heart disease, make sure your cardiologist knows what you're up to. You may not be a candidate for PDE5 inhibitors if you are taking certain heart medications.

Read the fine print. Like all prescription medicines, PDE5 inhibitors have a long list of possible side effects. Read the fine print describing the possible side effects before taking the pill and take care if you develop any symptoms. In addition, look out for newer drugs, like avanafil from VIVUS, Inc., that reportedly work faster and have fewer side effects.

Try, try again. If you've tried a PDE5 inhibitor and it failed, it doesn't necessarily mean that it can't be the solution to your problem. It could be that you just aren't using the drug properly or your doctor doesn't have the dosage right yet.

All three versions of this type of drug, more or less, work the same way, but they each have their particular quirks. For example, taking

Viagra after eating a heavy meal can weaken its effectiveness. They also have different "staying power." Viagra and Levitra are good for about four hours. Cialis has a window of 24 to 36 hours, making it more convenient for spontaneous or repetitive sex. Which drug is most appropriate for you is something to discuss with your doctor.

Viva Viagra!

It was the early 1990s and scientists from U.S.-based Pfizer Inc. were working with a group of men in the United Kingdom on a promising new drug to correct the blood flow problem associated with high blood pressure and angina. They gave the drug the code name UK-92480.

After months and months of testing, hope was fading. The drug, a synthetic chemical compound called sildenafil citrate, looked like a dud — it was doing nothing to improve blood flow in its test patients. In a last-ditch effort, the researchers decided to increase the dosage and see what would happen. It increased blood flow all right, but not particularly to the patients' hearts. It caused them to have erections — and some of the men hadn't had one in years.

For Pfizer it was like hitting the lottery. The accidental discovery became the first drug that could help men experience an erection strong enough to do the job. When the FDA finally approved it in 1998 it was an instant success. It soon became the butt of late-night talk show jokes and prompted countless questions from small children watching TV commercials: "Mommie, what's ED?"

Be careful where you buy. Viagra, Cialis, and Levitra are expensive, which prompts some men to purchase them more cheaply over the Internet from countries outside of the United States. Be forewarned —

counterfeit erectile dysfunction drugs are big business and risky to your health. Studies have found that a significant number of prescription erectile dysfunction drugs sold online are completely bogus or contain toxic materials, incorrect proportions of active and inactive ingredients, and inaccurate dosages. So stay on the safe side and deal only with a doctor and pharmacist you can trust.

Get your doctor to write you a note. A lot of insurance companies will not cover the cost of these drugs. Your doctor may be able to sway your insurance company by writing a letter explaining your medical circumstances.

Remember, drugs are not miracle workers. These drugs only go into action as a result of sexual stimulation. If there's no spark, it's not going to work.

Vasodilators: erection by injection

Before there was Viagra, there was a group of drugs called vasodilators that did the job of making an erection just as effectively as modern medication. The only hitch is that these drugs are not taken by mouth; they are injected directly into the penis. Vasodilators are an option — albeit an inconvenient one — for men who have lost nerve function and are not candidates for PDE5 inhibitors.

In reality, the idea of self-injecting medication into your penis is no different from giving yourself a shot — or getting one from a nurse, for that matter — anywhere else on the body. It's a quick, prickly sensation that goes away in a flash.

The experience begins in your doctor's office where he will do a few experiments to find the correct mix and strength of drugs that will give you an erection any time you want. Over the decades, researchers have found different vasodilators work in different ways. These days most doctors use a combination of three different drugs — papaverine (Pavabid), phentolamine (Regitine), and alprostadil (Caverject).

After the right dosage is determined, the doctor will teach you how to use a hypodermic needle and inject the medication into the base of your penis. You'll begin by practicing with a doll and then on yourself. An alternative to the shot is to insert a tiny tube into the urethra and drop in a pellet containing alprostadil. It takes about five to 20 minutes for the drugs to take effect, but it requires sexual stimulation to really take notice.

Vasodilators work by relaxing the smooth muscle and dilating blood vessels so blood can engorge the penis. They circumvent the job of the prostatic nerves, so they can be an effective treatment for men whose nerves are no longer intact.

Researchers are currently testing vasodilators to see if regular injections, whether accompanied by intercourse or not, can promote the return of normal erections if treatment is begun shortly after surgery.

The downside of the treatment is that your erection may not automatically go away at the expected time. Also, over time the treatment can cause scarring. A dose that's too large can cause priapism, an erection that can last for several hours. In addition to the awkward situation this poses, priapism is painful and dangerous. Left untreated, it can damage penile tissue. An injection of an adrenaline-like drug into the penis will resolve the problem.

Another downside is that vasodilators only have about a 70 percent success rate. In some cases blood vessels are just too damaged for the medication to overcome. While they work at the outset, blood engorgement can be diverted from the penis before intercourse.

About 500,000 men a year are game to give the medication a try, and about half of them are satisfied enough to continue it long term. Some men just don't like injecting themselves in the penis and find the shots uncomfortable. Some men complain that the pellets cause burning.

Like oral medication, penile injections are expensive, about $7 a shot. As with PDE5 inhibitors, a letter from your doctor to your insurance company might help if coverage is an issue.

Vacuum pump: inflation at its best

If needling your penis is too extreme, you can pump it up with a vacuum erection device (VED). It has been found to do the job when other methods fail, no matter what physical problem is causing impotence.

The VED, which has been around for 50 years, is an airtight acrylic tube fitted with a constricting ring and attached to a pump. Here's how it works. Just before intercourse, you place the tube over the penis and start pumping. You can do this by hand, though some more expensive models are electrically powered. The pumping action creates negative air pressure in the tube, which causes the vessels in the penis to fill with blood, just like a normal erection.

Once the erection is strong — it takes just a few minutes — you slip off the constricting ring at the bottom of the tube and slide it to the base of the penis to prevent blood from seeping back out. You pop off the tube and you're ready for love. The device is good to keep an erection for about a half-hour. If the constricting ring is left on too long, it can damage the penis.

From a medical point of view, the VED is the best solution for men who don't respond to drug therapy. As long as the device is used properly, there should be no risk of serious side effects, and it can be used as often as desired.

For all its technical effectiveness, only about 50 percent of men find it an acceptable solution. Many couples don't like the interruption it brings to lovemaking, and some men complain that the constricting ring is uncomfortable. Some men also don't like what it does to the penis. After use, the penis can go numb, become discolored, and feel cold to the touch.

The device is available by medical prescription and runs between $200 and $500.

Surgery: the main squeeze

You've surely heard of and may have seen silicon-implanted breasts. So why not a silicon-implanted erection! If no other solution works for you or isn't appealing, then a surgically implanted erection is a possible, though extreme, solution.

The penile prosthesis is a hydraulic system consisting of two hollow, flexible cylinders that are implanted in the penis; a fluid-filled reservoir that goes in the lower abdomen; and a squeezable pump that is inserted in the scrotum. When the time is right, you manually squeeze the pump in the scrotum, which releases the fluid. After a few squeezes the rods snap to attention. Presto! You have an erection. Later, you press a valve at the top of the pump, and the fluid goes back into the reservoir. The rods deflate, and the erection dies.

There is another, less complicated version based on the same principle. It involves implanting a spring-loaded rod in the penis, that is like having a permanent erection. It folds the penis in close to the body so it does not appear obvious. When you're ready for intercourse, you bend it into an erect position.

Though it sounds extreme, the entire surgery is managed with one 2-inch incision and takes about two hours. It can be performed on an outpatient basis or may require an overnight stay in the hospital. However, you'll have to wait about six weeks before taking it on a test drive. The surgery carries the same serious risks as any surgery involving an open incision and anesthesia.

Even though it is considered the most extreme solution for impotence, it doesn't work for every man. Men who have had radiation therapy in the pelvic area or have a compromised immune system may not qualify.

The test you can sleep through

You can't always assume your impotence is the fault of your faulty prostate. Doctors have a procedure called the nocturnal penile tumescence and rigidity (NPTR) test that can figure it out, but you have to spend the night in a sleep lab while a technician observes for movement under the covers. However, you can do the test on your own in the privacy of your own bedroom.

The NPTR tests for the presence of a nocturnal erection. Testosterone levels peak around daybreak, which can cause an erection. Almost every man experiences it. Also, an erection can occur during the deep sleep cycle called rapid eye movement, or REM, sleep. Either way, if you are able to get an erection in your sleep, the cause of your impotence is not structural.

Your inability to have an erection is likely related to low testosterone levels at other times. You might benefit from supplementation with a prescription testosterone gel, such as AndroGel. If you are capable of having nocturnal erections, you may also benefit from taking drugs that increase blood flow to the penis such as Viagra or, perhaps, with a lesser benefit, by taking niacin.

The home test is easy. All that's required is a roll of perforated stamps. Adhere the roll to your flaccid penis at bedtime. If you have an erection while you're asleep, your inflating penis will snap the perforations. You'll know in the morning if you physically have what it takes to achieve an erection. If you find the stamps intact, don't fret yet. Keep trying for a few more nights.

Part 3

The prostate protection plan

The prostate-protecting lifestyle: live like an ancient Greek

Let's suppose you're on active surveillance for early-stage prostate cancer and your doctor tells you there's a significant chance that you could delay treatment indefinitely on your own, without medication or other medical intervention, by making simple and healthy changes in your lifestyle. Suppose your doctor says these changes would actually enhance the way you feel, the way you look, and your outlook on life. Would you do it?

Or, let's say you're a man with an enlarged prostate struggling with lower urinary tract problems who desperately doesn't want to deal with the side effects of drugs, but also doesn't look forward to the agony and inconvenience of always having a vision of a bathroom foremost in mind. Suppose your doctor tells you that you could diminish your symptoms, and the size of your prostate might even shrink all on its own, by making many of the same simple and healthy lifestyle changes. Would you do it?

Now, let's say you're a man with a family history of prostate cancer. You live your life ignoring your prostate because as sure as shootin' you know you're going to get cancer and maybe even die from it.

But what if you found out that your genes are not your destiny — that it's now been proven that these genes may be kept dormant and suppressed from ever causing you any harm, if you simply choose the right lifestyle. Would you want to find out what that lifestyle is and follow it?

The sensible answer to all these questions is of course. Nevertheless, there is that nagging fear that doing "what's good for you" is going to ruin the life you love and make you miserable. There is also a nagging suspicion that it's just all going to be a waste of time. Well, put those fears and suspicions aside. There is an encouraging consensus among many specialists that the health of your prostate, to a great degree, is in your own control.

Experts say that as much as 90 percent of prostate trouble is created by your own environment — eating too much of the wrong foods and not enough of the right ones, sitting too long in a chair, spending too much time idle or driving when you should be active and walking, allowing too much stress in your life and not getting enough sleep, and being bombarded with toxins that oxidize your cells, compromise your immune system, and make you vulnerable to disease.

There is mounting evidence that these factors, which are largely under your control, greatly influence prostate health and the growth of prostate cells, and help determine if cancer cells will remain harmless and inconsequential or advance to a threatening stage. The fact is, there would be a lot less prostate trouble in the world if modern man could just learn to live life a little differently.

Ancient thinking

Hippocrates, an ancient Greek and the Father of Medicine, preached that good health and healing come from a good diet, plenty of physical exercise, clean fresh air, and a good night's sleep.

Back to the 60s: the retro-Grecian formula

Everything modern researchers now know about the relationship between prostate disease and a healthy lifestyle would come as no surprise to "ancient" Greeks. Not the Greeks of the classical age, but some very long-lived Greeks who were born more than 70 years ago on the sunny isle of Crete, just south of mainland Greece.

Though many of the islands nestled in this part of the world have made room for large tourist resorts and adopted many Western habits, much of the older population of Crete has managed to keep its old-fashioned ways. Among them is their daily ritual of gathering in the open air at a rural taverna to enjoy good food, drink, and camaraderie after a long day working the land. In short, they like to eat, drink, and have fun just like the rest of us.

Yet, there is something decidedly different in their approach to "the good life." You won't see them arriving by car. Mostly they show up on foot or bicycle. You won't find them standing at a bar, drinking away the stress of the day. You won't find evidence of traffic jams, text messaging, or multi-tasking. What you'd find, should you visit there, is older, healthy, and happy men relaxing and enjoying themselves and each other in the clean, fresh air. There's no stress, no rush. Just good conversation and moderate drink around a table of food — one bearing the true fruits and vegetables of their daily labor.

Cretans enjoy one of the lowest prostate disease rates in the world, something that has been fascinating scientists since the end of World War II. Researchers back then also noticed that men in other areas of the Mediterranean Basin — France, Italy, Spain, Morocco, Tunisia, and Turkey — also had lower rates of prostate disease, particularly cancer.

In the last 70 years, hundreds of studies have been conducted on the lifestyle habits of multiple generations living in these Mediterranean nations to try to determine the secret to their good health. As the years passed by and more and more nations started to imitate American ways, researchers started to notice a startling shift in the incidence of prostate disease. It had them wondering: Could it have something to do with the modern way of life in developed countries?

Secrets of the Mediterranean

Today the Mediterranean Diet is known worldwide as perhaps the healthiest diet on the planet. While much of the focus has been on the diet's ability to stave off heart disease, there is plenty of convincing evidence showing that Mediterranean cuisine also promotes a healthy prostate.

The term Mediterranean Diet, however, is somewhat of a misnomer, because it implies that all nations along the Mediterranean eat the same way. This is not the case. Just as countries in this area celebrate different cultures, they also enjoy different cuisines. Back when research started, these differences were subtle. But starting around 1960, when air travel started to pick up, Western influences gradually started to take hold in faraway places. Before long, a new dietary pattern started to take shape in many parts of the world, and not for the better.

The biggest changes were found in the European nations along the Mediterranean. The French were eating more meat and butter. Italians and Spaniards maintained their love of fruits, vegetables, and olive oil, but dietary patterns changed in every other way. Almost everywhere people were eating more red meat and more dairy foods. The convenience of refined flour replaced whole grain. Hard liquor started appearing on bar shelves, causing a decline in wine consumption. Overall, total olive oil consumption dropped thirtyfold and consumption of fruits and vegetables dipped fivefold. Everywhere, that is, except a few places like rural Sardinia and Crete.

By the 1990s, researchers were documenting another shift. The closer a region got to adopting the Western style of living, the closer it got to the Western cancer rate. Today, the United States, Western Europe, Australia, and Canada have the highest rates of prostate disease and cancer in the world. It's estimated that one out of every six American men will someday get a diagnosis of prostate cancer and that most older men have some degree of prostate cancer.

There is a great deal of evidence showing that prostate disease, to a large degree, is driven by the Western style of eating and living. When the International Association of Cancer Research (IACR) last examined the world's scientific findings on what is known to cause and prevent cancer, the researchers concluded that the incidence of the world's leading killing cancers would dramatically decline if people adopted a healthier style of living.

These cancers, the IACR concluded, are lifestyle cancers, led in the United States by lung cancer, associated with smoking, and followed by prostate and colorectal cancers. The IACR also concluded that if people throughout the world replaced the Western diet and sedentary habits with a lifestyle more akin to the ancient Greeks, the rate of killer cancers would dramatically decline.

How to avoid prostate surgery

When it comes to avoiding surgery for prostate cancer, positive lifestyle changes can make a difference. That's what well-known diet and heart disease researcher Dean Ornish, M.D., discovered when he found a group of men on active surveillance for early-stage prostate cancer willing to volunteer for a lifestyle makeover.

For the experiment Dr. Ornish randomly assigned the men into an intensive lifestyle regimen that included a vegan diet, nutritional supplements, moderate daily exercise, and a stress reduction program. Dr. Ornish described the diet as "intensive, but palatable and practical" — proven by the volunteers' 95 percent adherence to the program.

After one year, the men on the Ornish program achieved a "statistically significant" reduction in PSA levels. The closer the men adhered to the program, the greater was their improvement in PSA. A second group of men, who were also on active surveillance but were not following the program, experienced an average 6 percent *increase* in PSA.

What was more dramatic, however, is what Dr. Ornish found when he extracted blood serum from both groups of men and fed it to cancer cells in a petri dish. The cancer cells that were fed serum from the men who were *not* on the Ornish program grew eight times faster than the cells fed serum from men on the program.

> On the Ornish diet, cancer cells almost stopped growing.

Here's what the Ornish prostate program looked like.

- A vegan diet — meaning no food from animals, including eggs, cheese, and milk — consisting of a daily serving of tofu, 2 ounces of fortified soy protein mixed into a beverage, vegetables, fruits, legumes, and whole grains. Daily intake was limited to 10 percent of calories from fat.

- Exercise, including no less than 30 minutes of walking six days a week.

- A stress management program that included gentle yoga, meditation, stretching, controlled breathing, and progressive relaxation.

- A supplement regimen consisting of 3 grams of fish oil, 2 grams of vitamin C, 400 International Units (IU) of vitamin E, and 200 micrograms of selenium.

The prostate-protecting lifestyle

The description of a prostate-protecting lifestyle looks like this: A thin, nonsmoking, physically active man who eats red meat sparingly — if at all — gets plenty of exercise, avoids stress, drinks moderately — preferably wine —and consumes a daily diet with moderate amounts of complex carbohydrates, olive oil, fish, and enough fruits and vegetables to sustain high levels of prostate-protecting nutrients.

You can ease your way into this kind of lifestyle by gradually making modifications in the way you live — eating less steak and fewer burgers a week, using your feet or a bicycle instead of driving a couple of times a week, and learning to slow down, bit by bit. Studies show that making meaningful changes work better and become habit when you introduce them gradually instead of trying to abruptly change your life all at once. So, let's take a look, one by one, at the measures you can take to help protect your prostate.

Protection that lasts and lasts and . . .

Research shows that when people migrate to a new country and adopt their new country's diet and lifestyle habits, they also develop the country's cancer risk. There appears to be one exception: Greek men.

At least that's what Australian researchers concluded when they looked at the rate of prostate cancer among men who emigrated from Greece, where the prostate cancer rate is one of the lowest, to Australia, where the rate is one of the highest.

Despite acclimating to the Australian style of living, "Greek migrant men in Australia have retained their low risk for prostate cancer," noted the researchers. They could draw only one conclusion: Preference for the diet of their homeland continued to bestow benefits in the present.

Eat like an ancient Greek

As is typical in research, scientists started to study the lifestyle of people in Crete and other Mediterranean countries by examining their diet and dissecting it one food at a time. They found the fruits and vegetables grown in the Mediterranean's sunny climes are abundant in cancer-fighting polyphenols. Olive oil is superior in good-for-you monounsaturated fat. Wine is a unique reservoir of activated, health-enhancing resveratrol. The fish and seafood that swim the Mediterranean and become a meal almost daily contain important heart- and prostate-protecting omega-3 fatty acids. The daily custom of eating homemade breads provides important and nourishing fiber.

As research accumulated, scientists discovered that many of these foods are protective against many diseases — prostate disease, heart disease, cancer, Alzheimer's, Parkinson's disease. And the list keeps on growing.

A few years ago, researchers from the University of Florence in Italy examined the cumulative effect of 12 major studies conducted during the prior decade on 1.5 million lifelong residents of Crete. They concluded that their good health is not coming from just one food, but from a variety of foods. They believe the foods that comprise the Cretan diet most likely work synergistically to build a fortress against the insults that lead to chronic disease. "The greater the adherence to the Mediterranean diet, the greater the reduction in occurrence and mortality" of chronic disease, such as cancer and heart disease, the researchers noted in their study.

An American study that same year on the dietary habits of 25,623 Greeks came to the same conclusion: The Mediterranean Diet as a whole is more protective against all forms of cancer than any one food or group of foods or nutrients. But it is the Cretan diet, in particular, that deserves the credit for bestowing especially good prostate health, noted urology expert Allison Hodge, M.D., in the journal *Molecular Nutrition and Food Research*. The Cretan diet offers just a little bit more of what makes the Mediterranean diet so healthy, such as:

- more vegetables, particularly wild plants

- more fruit — it's the preferred dessert

- lots of nuts and olives

- heavy use of olive oil

- whole grains, mostly in the form of bread rather than pasta

- more cheese, but less milk

- more fish

- less meat

- wine in moderation, usually as part of the meal

You'll find the specifics of these and other prostate-friendly foods and nutrients in the next two chapters.

Remember, what's good for the heart is good for the prostate

Cancer is the second leading cause of death in American men next to heart disease, but heart disease is the undisputed number one cause of death in men who have prostate cancer. So does that mean there is a correlation between prostate cancer and heart disease? The answer is yes, according to research at University of Michigan Medical Center. Any effort you make to reduce heart disease is also reducing your risk of prostate disease.

Both prostate cancer and benign prostatic hyperplasia (BPH) have characteristics in common with heart disease — obesity, lack of physical activity, high cholesterol, high blood sugar, high blood pressure, and a high-fat diet. "Patients need to know that a heart-healthy lifestyle is also a prostate-healthy lifestyle," the Michigan researchers concluded in their study, published in *The American Journal of Medicine*.

When the World Health Organization examined the lifestyle habits of populations in 52 countries, they concluded that if people could control nine risk factors, the cumulative effect would add up to a spectacular 90 percent reduction in the incidence of heart disease. That means that the cause of heart disease is only 10 percent beyond our control. Controlling these risk factors would mean:

- no tobacco use.

- maintaining low total cholesterol that includes keeping dangerous LDL cholesterol below 100.

- maintaining normal blood pressure.

- keeping weight normal and body mass index in the low 20s.

- maintaining normal blood sugar in the absence of diabetes.

- getting a minimum of 30 minutes of physical exercise every day.

- eating large amounts of fruits and vegetables every day.

- drinking alcohol in moderation.

- avoiding depression.

So be diligent in all things heart-smart. If it's good for your heart, you know it's got to be good for the prostate.

Watch your weight — go down

If you could do but one thing to protect your prostate from potential or advancing disease, most doctors, hands down, would tell you to maintain a healthy weight. Research shows that being overweight or obese increases the risk of BPH and prostate cancer. Studies also show that men who are overweight and overeat are increasing their chance of getting aggressive prostate cancer, the type that kills.

If you have prostate cancer and are overweight, losing excess fat is particularly important because research shows it can help slow the disease's progression — something important for guys on active surveillance to keep in mind. Researchers believe that obesity contributes to prostate disease because it messes with the delicate balance of hormones involved in fueling prostate disease, including testosterone, estrogen, and insulin, the hormone that regulates blood sugar.

The standard doctors use these days to establish healthy weight is body mass index (BMI), which compares height to weight to estimate the ratio of body fat to lean muscle. However, it does not measure actual body fat. So if you're a body builder or you work out a lot, your BMI could reflect your muscle mass more than it does body fat. Nevertheless, a high BMI is still associated with a higher risk of prostate cancer.

Guidelines define normal weight as a BMI of 19 to 24. Overweight is a BMI of 25 to 29, obesity is a BMI between 30 and 39, and extreme obesity is considered a BMI of 40 or greater. A BMI under 19 is considered underweight.

Height	Normal weight BMI: 19-24	Overweight BMI: 25-29	Obese BMI: 30-39
5'6"	118-148	155-179	186-241
5'7"	121-153	159-185	191-249
5'8"	125-158	164-190	197-256
5'9"	128-162	169-196	203-263
5'10"	132-167	174-202	209-271
5'11"	136-172	179-208	215-279
6'	140-177	184-213	221-287
6'1"	144-182	189-219	227-295
6'2"	148-186	194-225	233-303

Studies show that men with a BMI of 30 or greater have an 80 percent greater risk of developing prostate cancer than men with a BMI of less than 23. Studies also show that a body mass index of 30 and above increases your risk of dying from advanced prostate cancer.

Figuring out BMI takes a bit of arithmetic. It is calculated by multiplying your weight in pounds by 703, then dividing the result by your height in inches squared. Or, you can just use this chart. If you do not find your weight, calculate it to the closest number. For example, if you are 5 feet 6 inches tall and weigh 149, consider yourself on the high end of normal. If you're 154 pounds, you're on the low end of overweight.

Watch your waist — get leaner

Though BMI is considered important, what you're carrying around the middle is more important. A potbelly boosts your risk of getting prostate cancer, studies show. It also contributes to the woes associated with BPH. Men who have BPH and are too wide around the middle have more trouble controlling lower urinary tract problems and are more likely to end up needing the most extreme treatment — a radical prostatectomy to remove the prostate.

One study of nearly 26,000 men with BPH found a relationship between the severity of lower urinary tract symptoms and the amount of abdominal fat. They found that men with a waist measuring 43 inches or greater were most likely to have symptoms severe enough to necessitate surgery, while men with a waist 35 inches or smaller experienced the least severe symptoms.

Men have a small amount of estrogen-like female hormones in their bodies, just as women generally have a small amount of androgen or male hormones. A small amount of androgen can help spark sexual desire in women. Post-menopausal women or those who have had hysterectomies often will have more sexual interest if a very small amount of testosterone is added to estrogen replacement therapy. This generally doesn't produce masculine side effects.

However, higher than normal amounts of estrogen in a man have the opposite effect, dampening sexual desire and causing impotence. Fat, especially belly fat, actually makes estrogen-like molecules.

Researchers believe belly fat, especially, upsets the estrogen-to-testosterone ratio, which increases the risk of impotence and makes BPH worse.

Doctors calculate abdominal fat by measuring waist-to-hip ratio. The cutoff that divides risk from no risk is 0.8. Finding your hip-to-waist ratio is easy. Stand naked and relaxed — no pulling in the gut! — and, with a tape measure, first measure your waist just above the navel and then your hips at the widest part. Divide your waist measurement by your hip measurement. For example, a 38-inch waist divided by 36-inch hips equals close to 1.

Having surgery? Stay trim

Men who gain five or more pounds prior to a radical prostatectomy for prostate cancer are more than twice as likely to have a recurrence of the disease, according to a study involving 1,337 men who underwent surgery at Johns Hopkins Medical Center.

"We surveyed men whose cancer was confined to the prostate and surgery should have cured most of them, yet some cancers recurred," said Corinne Joshu, Ph.D., one of the researchers in the study. "Obesity and weight gain may be factors that tip the scale to recurrence."

The men reported their weight and physical activity five years before and one year after their surgery.

The study found that men who gained about five pounds prior to surgery had twice the rate of recurrence compared to men whose weight remained stable.

Get a move on

It's no revelation that the more active you are, the better off you are in terms of many aspects of life — your heart health, your longevity, your physical appearance, and your happiness. What you don't hear much about is how important exercise is to your prostate.

More than a dozen studies have found that regular exercise can help reduce the chances of developing prostate cancer and BPH. The reason? Exercise helps keep hormones in balance. Exercise improves the ratio of estrogen to testosterone, says *The Physician and Sports Medicine*. It also helps keep insulin and another substance called insulin-like growth factor — both of which are implicated in prostate cancer — in check. Plus, exercise helps you control your weight and keep your waistline trim.

Two Harvard Medical School studies involving more than 3,000 men found that the frequency and level of heart-pumping aerobic exercise correlated to reducing the risk of developing fatal prostate cancer. One study found that men who exercised aerobically for a half-hour a day, or three or more hours a week, reduced their risk of dying from prostate cancer by 35 percent. Men who walked four or more hours a week reduced their risk by 23 percent.

Other research indicates that black men, who are genetically at greatest risk for prostate cancer, can cut their risk significantly with frequent and regular moderate to vigorous exercise starting at a young age.

If you have BPH, exercise can help diminish lower urinary tract symptoms. A study of nearly 3,000 men with BPH found that moderate to vigorous physical exercise resulted in stronger urine flow and a diminished sensation that the bladder was not completely empty. The men also reported less need to get up in the middle of the night to urinate. The men who worked out the hardest reported getting the most symptom relief.

So how much exercise is considered optimum for prostate protection? Five or more hours a week of vigorous activity, say researchers from the Harvard School of Public Health. This includes such things as jogging, rowing, cycling, or playing tennis or squash. However, they noted, any amount of exercise is better than no exercise at all. Even 15 minutes a day was found to reduce prostate cancer risk in some men.

Find the path of most resistance

Lifting weights, in and of itself, does not reduce the incidence of prostate disease, but having good muscle mass is important if you have prostate cancer, and it is crucial if you're being treated with hormone deprivation therapy.

Muscle mass is fueled by testosterone, so when hormone production is cut off, as it is with hormone therapy, muscle mass starts to decline, and it can happen rapidly. The result is loss of strength, lethargy, and weight gain. Resistance training, however, can help counteract these effects. "A relatively brief exposure to exercise significantly improved muscle mass, strength, physical function, and balance," Australian researchers reported in the *Journal of Clinical Oncology* after putting men undergoing hormone deprivation therapy for prostate cancer on a resistance training program.

Resistance training is also important to men who choose to go through the two-month course of daily radiation treatments for prostate cancer. Researchers, reporting in the same journal, found a combination of strength training and aerobic exercise helped increase stamina in men undergoing the treatment. Physical fitness, they found, is important in mitigating fatigue, building strength, resisting weight gain, and generally improving the quality of life for men undergoing cancer treatment.

Get a special perk from a physically intense job

When it comes to prostate health, men who have jobs involving physical labor have one up on desk jockeys, according to two studies.

One study followed men working in the aerospace industry in Southern California over the course of 40 years. The researchers found prostate cancer developed more frequently in men who had sedentary jobs, such as administrators, managers, analysts, and engineers, than in men whose jobs required a high level of continuous activity, such as mechanics, patrolmen, electricians, truck-lift operators, welders, and janitors.

Another broader study examined men from different lines of work. The researchers divided the jobs into five categories according to the physical intensity of the job: sedentary, light in physical labor, moderately laborious, high in physical labor, and very high in physical labor. They found that men who spent their careers doing the most physically intense work had the lowest rate of prostate cancer and men in sedentary jobs had the highest rate of prostate cancer. Risk went down with the physical intensity of the job.

As with exercise, the researchers speculate that men who are physically active during the daytime are better able to keep male hormones in balance, which lowers the risk of prostate problems. If you have a sedentary job, doctors suggest compensating for the lack of daytime activity by engaging in physical activity during lunch and taking short walks during breaks.

Salut! Make a toast to the prostate

Drinking, even moderately, has been associated with higher rates of cancer, but numerous population studies have not been able to find a link between moderate drinking and prostate cancer, either pro or con. However, a lower rate of benign prostatic hyperplasia (BPH) is associated with alcohol consumption.

A total of 14 studies involving 120,091 men revealed a "significantly decreased likelihood of benign prostatic hyperplasia or lower urinary tract symptoms with increased alcohol intake," reported researchers from the University of California, San Diego and the VA Medical

Center San Diego in La Jolla, who compiled that data. Compared to men who didn't drink at all, consumption of about 1.2 ounces of alcohol a day — equal to around half an ounce of pure alcohol — was associated with a 35 percent decreased risk of BPH. There is also evidence, though it is not consistent, that drinking can reduce urinary problems in men who already have BPH.

Researchers believe alcohol has a positive effect on BPH and its symptoms because it has a beneficial effect on the production and metabolism of testosterone.

Note, however, that half an ounce is about the amount of alcohol in one beer or a small glass of wine. Moderate drinking, which is defined as no more than two drinks a day for a man (and one a day for a woman), is promoted by the American Heart Association as having health benefits because it is associated with a lower risk of cardiovascular disease. However, nothing good can be said for heavy drinking, especially when it comes to many forms of cancer. And that includes prostate cancer.

Though moderate alcohol consumption neither increases nor reduces the risk of prostate cancer, heavy drinking has a detrimental affect. When doctors at the National Cancer Institute examined the alcohol habits of 295,000 men, they found that heavy drinking, defined as six or more drinks a day, increased the risk of prostate cancer by 25 percent. Men who drank three to six alcoholic beverages a day had a 19 percent greater risk for the cancer. Risk dropped to 6 percent for men who drank three drinks a day.

Bottom line: If you don't drink, don't start. If you do drink, limit consumption to two drinks a day, and make it beer or wine. As you'll read in the next chapters, both contain nutrients that may help promote prostate health.

Don't burn the midnight oil

Researchers sometimes look for environmental causes of disease in creative ways. One such instance is the lifestyle habit of staying up late at night. It appears that there may be a connection between exposure to artificial light and a high risk for prostate cancer.

A joint study by researchers at the University of Connecticut and the University of Haifa found that countries with the highest levels of artificial light at night have the highest rates of prostate cancer. For the study, researchers gathered data from 164 countries on their level of nighttime illumination and electricity consumption and adjusted them by the geographic distribution of the population of each country in order to accurately measure "the amount of artificial light per night per person."

"At the very first stage of the study, it already became clear that there is a marked link between the incidence of prostate cancer and levels of nighttime artificial illumination and electricity consumption," says Richard Stevens, Ph.D., of the University of Connecticut.

For the next stage of the study, the researchers isolated the amount of artificial light at night per person in order to examine its effect. The countries were divided into three groups: those with little exposure to light at night, those with medium exposure, and those with high exposure. They found that men in countries with medium exposure to artificial light had an incidence of prostate cancer 30 percent greater than men in countries with the lowest exposure. Men living in countries with the highest exposure to artificial light had an incidence of prostate cancer 80 percent higher than those living in countries with the lowest exposure.

Where does the United States fit in? At the highest level, of course.

Dr. Stevens suggests a number of theories that could explain why exposure to artificial light increases the incidence of prostate cancer. Artificial light interferes with the secretion of melatonin, a brain hormone that controls the sleep cycle; it interferes with the body's circadian rhythms, or biological clock, because artificial light mimics natural daylight; and it compromises the immune system, making it easier for cancer cells to manifest and grow.

This isn't the first time that scientists linked disruption of the day and night cycle to cancer. One study involving more than 100,000 female nurses found that those who worked the night shift had a higher incidence of breast cancer. Another study involving flight attendants whose internal biological clocks were upset by travel on transatlantic flights produced similar results.

Relax while changing your diet

There's good stress — the kind that gets you pumped up and leads to great achievement or just personal satisfaction — and there's bad stress — the kind that leads to nothing but mental fatigue, a depressed immune system, and chronic health problems, such as prostate cancer.

Recently, researchers at the Moores Cancer Center and School of Medicine at the University of California, San Diego wanted to find out if reducing the stress that comes with switching to a healthy diet, impacted the spread of prostate cancer.

Their study had men with recurrent prostate cancer eat more whole grains, cruciferous and leafy green vegetables, beans, legumes, and fruit. Plus, they were told to eat less meat, fewer dairy products, and cut back on refined carbohydrates. Although there's already a lot of evidence that says switching to a plant-based diet can lower the risk of prostate cancer progressing, many men find this a difficult and stressful thing to do. And, as you've learned, stress is not good for your emotional or physical health.

That's why they were also coached in ways to control these feelings of stress — through activities like yoga, tai chi, and time spent in quiet thought. It took just 15 minutes a day, but the results were considered spectacular. PSA levels dropped in these healthy eaters who learned how to reduce stress, and the average PSA doubling time increased from about one year to more than nine years.

In addition to adopting healthier eating habits, try any or all of these simple lifestyle strategies to help reduce your own stress.

- Get plenty of sleep.

- Laugh more.

- Exercise regularly.

- Stretch and relax your muscles.

- Play some music.

- Practice deep breathing exercises.

- Don't sit still for too long.

- Take a vacation.

- Engage in a relaxing hobby like gardening.

- Pray.

Snuff the cigarettes and cigars

There's nothing cool about smoking, if you value your life. It is a leading cause of heart disease. It is undeniably the leading cause of lung cancer, which kills more American men than any other cancer. And smoking appears to play a role in the second leading cause of cancer death in men — prostate cancer.

Smoking can increase your risk of prostate cancer by 50 percent, according to Sheila Weinmann, Ph.D., a researcher for the Center for Health and Research at Kaiser Permanente Northwest in Portland, Ore. She came to this conclusion after reviewing the medical records of 768 men at the center who died from prostate cancer. Studies have also found a relationship between smoking and a higher risk of BPH. One study, conducted by doctors at Johns Hopkins Medical Center, found that former heavy smokers had more urinary tract problems as a result of BPH than men who never smoked.

If you smoke, you probably agree with Mark Twain who said, "Giving up smoking is the easiest thing in the world. I know because I've done it thousands of times."

Like Mark Twain, you've probably tried to quit more times than you remember. An estimated 70 percent of the 1.3 billion people world-wide who smoke say they'd like to kick the habit but can't. If you're one of them, you may feel that the last thing you need is family and friends harassing you about smoking. However, harassment might be just what you need to stop smoking for good.

In one novel experiment, a group of researchers from North Dakota University recruited a group of volunteer student smokers to help with a campaign exploring the best ways to disseminate information on the consequences of smoking. The format they decided to use on the students was text messages and emails. The students were blasted with messages about the negative aspects of smoking, includ-ing how it causes bad breath, smelly clothes, wrinkles, yellow teeth, and lung cancer. Messages were sent out eight times a day for two weeks. Though the researchers never suggested the point of the study was to get the students to quit smoking, half of the students reported that the campaign motivated them to stop smoking.

Worry about the side effects of smoking was the motivating factor that led them to quit, reported the researchers. Therefore, comments about the undesirable social aspects of smoking may have more influence on kicking the habit than carping about health hazards.

Monogamous sex is the only true 'safe sex'

Sexually transmitted diseases do not cause prostate cancer, but they can cause inflammation of the prostate, and chronic inflammation increases the risk of prostate cancer. The risk of sexually transmitted disease goes up with participation in indiscriminate sex and with the number of sexual partners you have. Having a monogamous mar-riage is much healthier than alternative sexual lifestyles.

Doctors recommend using a condom if you are not in a monogamous relationship, but this isn't a foolproof method of preventing disease.

Foods that promote prostate health

One of the most enjoyable ways you can pamper your prostate is by feeding it well. Of all the lifestyle options associated with prostate health, experts concur, the biggest benefits come from making smart dietary choices.

Not only can certain foods help prevent prostate cancer, they can also help slow its progression and even help put it in remission. Avoiding the wrong foods can help prevent an enlarged prostate, and eating the right foods can help alleviate symptoms if you already have a problem. Healthy eating stokes the immune system, which can help fight off a prostate infection.

Making smart dietary choices can help you achieve other benchmarks associated with a prostate-protecting lifestyle. Foods that promote prostate health benefit the waistline. If you're overweight, they can help you to naturally lose weight and pull your belt in a few notches. The right food choices will also help give you the energy to get out and exercise, a lifestyle practice essential to prostate health.

There's no question that nutrition plays a central role in prostate health. For decades researchers have been studying the eating habits of populations around the world searching for dietary clues that put some people at high risk for prostate disease and help protect others. By using nutritionally controlled diets, food diaries, and dietary questionnaires as scientific tools, researchers have come to the conclusion that certain foods and food groups have a major influence on prostate health. Among some of the major findings:

- Diaries that detailed the food choices of more than 5,000 men participating in the long-term Prostate Cancer Prevention Trial showed that a diet low in saturated fat and red meat, high in protein and vegetables, and moderate in alcohol consumption was associated with a reduced risk of benign prostatic hyperplasia (BPH).

- A study involving more than 32,000 men with BPH found that men who ate the most vegetables suffered the least from lower urinary tract symptoms. They also were least likely to require surgery to find symptom relief.

- The best dietary protection against prostate cancer comes from reducing saturated fat, red meat, and processed foods and eating a diet focused on fish, soy foods, legumes, vegetables, nuts, and grains.

- A review of the diets of more than 175,000 men by the National Cancer Institute found a relationship between high consumption of red meat and processed food and the incidence of advanced prostate cancer.

- Studies show that men who regularly eat tomatoes, broccoli, cabbage, Brussels sprouts, and tofu and drink green tea can cut their risk of prostate cancer in half. However, don't overdo the tofu and other soy products such as texturized vegetable protein (TVP) that is added to many processed food products. Eating soy protein has been associated with sharply higher rates of dementia in one highly regarded study.

Nature knows best

When it comes to knowing what's best for you, man is no match for foods closer to those in the Garden of Eden. Man has given us salami, margarine, ice cream, processed cheese, and trans fats, and has refined the wholesomeness out of flours and grains — food processing that scientists believe contributes to prostate problems. Foods closer to those found in the preindustrial age are more likely to be a rich source of nutrition. Vegetables, whole grains, and fruits are all foods that come to the prostate's defense.

These foods contain much more than just the vitamins and minerals doctors say we need every day to sustain minimum health. Plant foods, especially those close to their wild cousins, contain a plethora of phytochemicals or phytonutrients, bioactive compounds that scientists have discovered offer extra nutritional value in the prevention and treatment of a wide variety of diseases. Scientists have identified thousands of them and believe there are thousands of others that have yet to be discovered. These nutrients vary widely in chemical structure and are categorized by the functions they perform. Flavones, carotenoids, phytoestrogens, and organosulfurs are but a few of the families of compounds associated with prostate health.

Some of these compounds have a special ability to stop the inflammatory process that damages cells and sets them off in a cancerous direction. Others have the ability to control hormones that instigate all types of prostate trouble. Many of them act as powerful antioxidants that defend cells from corrosion or boost the effectiveness of prostate-protecting vitamins and minerals or other phytonutrients.

Though there is no proof that certain foods you eat cause a troubled prostate, there is plenty of evidence that they contribute to it. Too much food from the butcher and processing plant and not enough from trees, vines, and the garden has created an imbalance in modern man's diet that is contributing to a diet too high in animal fat and too high in concentrated calories, both of which are incriminated in causing poor prostate health.

If you're a meat-and-potatoes kind of guy — and most American men are — the idea of doing without the foods you love probably is not sitting very well. So here's the good news. The goal isn't necessarily to do without; the goal is to do with less.

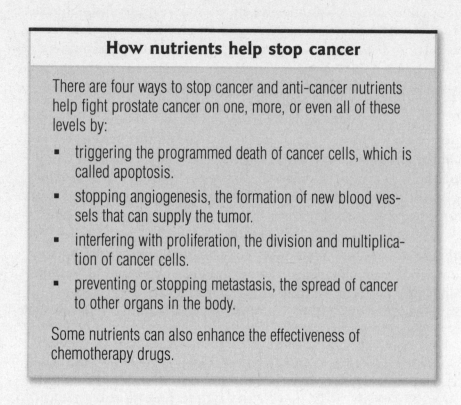

How nutrients help stop cancer

There are four ways to stop cancer and anti-cancer nutrients help fight prostate cancer on one, more, or even all of these levels by:

- triggering the programmed death of cancer cells, which is called apoptosis.

- stopping angiogenesis, the formation of new blood vessels that can supply the tumor.

- interfering with proliferation, the division and multiplication of cancer cells.

- preventing or stopping metastasis, the spread of cancer to other organs in the body.

Some nutrients can also enhance the effectiveness of chemotherapy drugs.

The pro-prostate eating style

There are no taboos. The pro-prostate eating style is all about minimizing dietary habits that lead to prostate disease and maximizing eating foods containing nutrients that have been found to enhance prostate health. Here are the guidelines based on what science knows about diet and the prostate.

Cut back on "bad" fat. It's not fat, per se, but the kind of fat you eat that incites prostate disease. And the instigator is saturated fat.

Saturated fat — the kind that comes from animal foods — is one of the leading suspects for creating a hostile nutritional environment in the prostate. Studies show it raises the risk of both BPH and prostate cancer.

A high saturated fat diet is a breeding ground for cancer cells. For example, when researchers fed test mice a diet consisting of 40 percent of calories mostly from saturated fat — about the same amount of fat consumed in the typical American man's diet — tumors grew twice as fast as tumors in mice fed a diet consisting of 21 percent of calories from fat. PSA levels were also highest in animals on the 40 percent fat rations.

In another study, researchers put test animals on a high-fat diet primarily of pork fat for 10 weeks to see how it would affect the prostate. Prostates started to enlarge in all of them. By contrast, animals fed a high-fat diet consisting of soybean and flaxseed oil did not experience prostate growth.

Here are a few ways you can cut back on harmful fat without much effort.

- Pare down a high-fat burger lunch by eliminating the cheese and fries on the side. Round out your lunch with a salad or vegetable-based soup instead.

- Stay away from creamy salad dressings and go for vinaigrette dressings. Always ask for your dressing on the side, but don't pour it on. Drizzle a small amount of the dressing onto your salad or dip your fork into the salad dressing and spear the greens.

- Dump the yolks from two of three eggs and have a three-egg breakfast with lots of whites.

- Do away with desserts except on special occasions. If you like to have dessert more often, opt for fresh fruit and dress it up with a dip of low-fat regular or frozen yogurt.

- Substitute a poached fruit topping for butter and maple syrup on pancakes.

- Avoid the deep fryer and turn to recipes for oven-fried foods that give you flavor without the fat.

- Bake French fries and make them crunchy by squirting them with a little olive oil.

- Ignore the deli counter at the supermarket and hit the salad bar instead. A rotisserie chicken can go a tasty long way as a healthier substitute for lunchmeats.

Make red meat a luxury. Red meat is a major contributor to the American male's high-fat diet. It is also one of the prostate's major enemies. The Prostate Cancer Prevention Trial found that men who ate five or more servings of red meat a week had a significantly higher risk of developing prostate cancer or BPH compared to men who ate red meat once a week. One study involving 6,000 men found that those who routinely consumed meat, eggs, milk, and cheese had a risk of fatal prostate cancer 3.6 times greater than men who rarely ate these foods.

If you're hooked on red meat, here are a few ways to help break the habit.

- Eat a salad several days a week for lunch instead of a burger.

- Have a chicken or turkey burger or sandwich instead of a sandwich made with beef or processed meats. Pile it high with vegetables, California-style.

- Share a steak when dining out and start with a big garden salad.

- Make one of your weekly meat meals a steak salad with thin slices of lean meat on top of a green salad.

- Chili con carne, with its bounty of beans and chilies, is good for you, but you can make it even better by substituting ground turkey for high-fat beef.

- Go vegetarian one day a week, then increase to two or more days a week.

Replace butter and margarine with healthy oils. Studies show a correlation between the amount of butter and margarine in the diet and the risk of BPH and prostate cancer. One study of 184 Greek men with BPH found one commonality in their diet: a preference for butter or margarine over olive oil. The study, reported in the journal *Urology*, found that increased consumption of butter or margarine was directly related to the risk of an enlarged prostate. By contrast, the researchers found no risk of enlargement in men who used olive oil as their fat of choice.

Grill carefully. Grilling or frying meats, poultry, and fish — though, not vegetables — produces a buildup of toxic chemicals called heterocyclic amines (HCAs) and polycyclic aromatic hydrocarbons (PAHs), well-known carcinogens that are readily absorbed when consumed. Traces of HCAs and PAHs have been found in human cancer cells, and population studies over the years have linked them to prostate cancer. They only start to build up at temperatures of 352 degrees. The higher the temperature and the longer the cooking time, the greater the toxic buildup.

Forget the milkshake. Studies consistently show that a diet high in dairy foods increases the risk of prostate cancer. Research in Sweden found that high consumption of dairy products was associated with a 50 percent greater risk of prostate cancer, including metastatic disease. A U.S. study that followed the diets of 20,805 men for 11 years found the risk was associated with consuming 2½ servings of dairy products a week. When researchers in Buffalo, N.Y. evaluated the diets of nearly 400 men with prostate cancer, they found that men who reported drinking three or more glasses of whole milk a day were at greatest risk compared to men who did not drink milk at all.

Milk is linked to prostate cancer for two reasons. One, it stimulates the production of insulin-like growth factor, a substance associated with prostate cancer. Also, milk contains phytanic acid, also found in red meat that is believed to feed cancer cells.

Trash the trans fats. When it comes to trans fats, the critics are harsh, many feeling they could quite possibly be the greatest health threat in our food supply.

There's no shortage of evidence that trans fats, found in man-made oils used to make packaged goods and fast foods, increase the risk of heart disease and heart attacks. Here's another reason to avoid them: They are just as bad for your prostate. A Canadian study that examined the nutrient content in the diets of more than 2,500 men concluded that men could significantly reduce their risk of prostate cancer simply by eliminating trans fats from their diets.

Stick with protein. A high-protein diet is associated with easing the lower urinary tract symptoms associated with BPH, according to results of the Prostate Cancer Prevention Trial. This is not a mixed message. There are a lot of ways to get protein other than by eating red meat and high-fat processed foods. Think skinless chicken and turkey, fish, pork tenderloin, legumes, nuts, and beans.

Become a more complex fellow. Consuming too many simple starches — like sugar and fiber-depleted white rice, white pasta, and white flour — and not enough complex carbohydrates — like high-fiber fruits, vegetables, and whole grains — is a bad combination. It produces higher levels of blood glucose and consequently higher levels of insulin necessary for the body to handle the glucose load. Several studies, including one involving more than 3,000 men in Italy, found that the higher the diet was in simple carbohydrates, the greater the risk of BPH.

These studies confirm what many researchers suspect: There is a relationship between high levels of insulin and prostate cancer. One study, conducted by the National Cancer Institute, found the risk of cancer was eight-and-a-half times greater in men with the highest insulin levels than in men with the lowest insulin levels.

Watch your cholesterol. Preliminary research suggests that a lifetime of eating a diet high in cholesterol might increase the risk of prostate cancer. Researchers came to this conclusion after a steady diet of high-cholesterol foods caused prostate tumors in test animals. The research, published in *The Journal of Urology*, suggests that cholesterol is harmful to the prostate because it increases testosterone levels. Also, cholesterol itself may be a slow-acting carcinogen that causes prostate tumors over time.

Go light on salt. Salt appears to aggravate lower urinary tract symptoms associated with BPH. In one study, scientists from the New England Research Institutes followed the dietary habits of nearly 2,000 Boston-area men with BPH for three years and found that those who ate the most salt in a day's time were twice as likely to experience more excruciating urinary tract symptoms. The difference amounted to 1,500 milligrams, or nearly a teaspoon, of salt a day!

Size back your portions. It's not just what you eat but how much you eat that counts. Studies show that heavy eaters have a risk of prostate cancer almost four times greater than men who eat more moderate portions. Not only is overeating associated with a higher risk of prostate cancer, but researchers at Johns Hopkins School of Medicine found a correlation between the number of calories consumed and the risk of developing high-grade prostate cancer.

Remembering the link between high levels of insulin and prostate cancer, experts suggest you eat smaller portions at meals to keep insulin at safe levels. This also helps to control weight, another risk factor.

Overeating is also implicated in BPH. In one study, men who kept their daily calorie count below 2,000 experienced few lower urinary tract troubles or none at all.

Portion control at mealtime happily permits eating healthy, low-calorie snacks between meals.

Count to nine daily. That would be nine servings of vegetables and fruits. Studies involving thousands of men suggest that you could cut your risk of prostate cancer in half and significantly reduce your chance of developing recurring cancer after prostate cancer treatment by eating more vegetables and less red meat.

The Prostate Cancer Prevention Trial found that men who ate the most vegetables had an 11 percent lower risk of developing BPH than men who ate the least number of vegetables.

For optimal prostate protection, most specialists recommend nine servings a day. However, it is not just quantity of vegetables that's important. Quality is also important, as you're about to find out.

Mediterranean gold

A diet rich in allium vegetables, olive oil, and tomatoes — the backbone of the Mediterranean diet — adds up to a reduced risk of prostate cancer, according to a study of nearly 1,000 men conducted in Australia.

The prostate-protecting food chain

The phytonutrients that promote prostate health exist in a wide array of plant foods, which is why a diet that emphasizes vegetables, fruits, and whole grains is so important. Some of these nutrients, however, are abundant and most active in certain foods. These are the foods scientists have identified that are especially prostate-friendly.

Alliums: garlic and onions head the 'A' team

"A" is for allium, a large family of culinary bulbs with a distinctive scent that sends an important message: Eating garlic and onions are good for your prostate.

This famous culinary couple, which plays an important role in Mediterranean cuisine, reigns over a kingdom of odiferous vegetables that arm the prostate with a unique weapon called allicin, which makes its presence known whenever it enters your air space.

Though garlic and onions each bring their own brand of chemistry to the health front, studies suggest they perform even better when they work as a team. For example, one study that followed the eating habits of nearly 4,000 men in Italy found that those who enjoyed eating onions and garlic had a reduced risk of an enlarged prostate compared to men who enjoyed either one or the other alone.

All alliums, however, are good for the prostate. One large study conducted in China found that men who had the highest combined consumption of alliums — either garlic, onions, scallions, leeks, shallots, or chives — had a significantly lower risk of prostate cancer than men who ate little or no alliums.

. . . and the winner is — the onion

The onion is an allium of unique distinction. As a stand-alone healer, the onion's reputation is well-documented, and not because it is the only food that can make a grown man cry. Onions possess more phytochemicals than any member of the allium clan and are the third richest source of cancer-fighting flavonols among all vegetables. (Broccoli and spinach are numbers one and two.) Also, onions are one of the few foods containing hydroxybenzoic acid, a special type of phytochemical that enhances the effectiveness of other antioxidants. Plus, they are a rare source of quercetin, another nutrient important to prostate health. Together, these nutrients are a warhorse of prostate protection. When researchers compared the biggest onion eaters to the biggest garlic eaters, they found that garlic reduced the risk of prostate cancer by 19 percent, but onions reduced it by 71 percent.

Onions get their signature tear-jerk reaction from allyl sulfate, a sulphur-smelling phytonutrient in allicin that is released when a knife slashes through its cells. The stronger the onion, the more sulphur, the higher the nutrient content. Of all the many varieties, yellow onions are the strongest and, therefore, possess the most prostate-protecting qualities. Vidalia onions, the sweetest and mildest variety, contain the least.

Experts say you can get prostate protection from eating onions as little as once or twice a week, but eating onions daily is best.

No-tears onions

You can keep allicin from reducing you to tears by refrigerating onions before peeling them. Cold slows the volatility of allicin, but does not destroy it. Though cutting onions under running water reduces tearing, it washes away allicin, meaning its prostate protection goes down the drain.

Garlic: two cloves a day

Alternative healers have been using garlic for decades to treat prostate cancer and bring relief for the symptoms of BPH.

Though thousands of population studies have been conducted on the therapeutic benefits of garlic, only a few of them have focused on prostate cancer. One study concluded that daily consumption of garlic can reduce the risk of prostate cancer by around 20 percent. Though other studies have been less positive, the National Cancer Institute considers the evidence strong enough to recommended eating two to three cloves of garlic a day.

(Also see *Aged Garlic Extract* on page 316.)

Smart advice for grill jockeys

Greeks traditionally eat meat sparingly. One of the most celebrated ways is as a grilled kabob of cubed lamb or veal laced between lots of vegetables. But, Greeks also like to grill, a cooking process that, along with frying, has been indicted as a prostate cancer-causing agent. Here's why.

Cooking and frying at high temperatures cause molecules in meat to break down and produce toxic substances called polycyclic aromatic hydrocarbons (PAHs). When consumed, these substances have the ability to induce DNA damage in cells. So it's not just red meat, or even the fat in meat, that's carcinogenic. It's also the cooking method that makes eating meat so risky — at least for most people, but not for Greeks. At least that's what one study found.

Greeks eat meat, but they don't seem to be affected by PAHs, a fact that caused Polish researchers to wonder: Is there something about their diet that is protecting Greeks from absorbing these harmful chemicals? The answer is, yes — fruits and vegetables.

According to the researchers, the rich polyphenol content of the fruits and vegetables commonly served with meat in the Mediterranean diet activates enzymes that scavenge the digestive system and zap these harmful compounds before they can do damage. "It's the proper ratio of vegetable to meat consumption that is responsible for cancer prevention," note the researchers — the perfect recipe for culinary detoxification.

The researchers didn't say exactly what that ratio should be, but think shish kabob — a long skewer containing not more than three or four small chunks of meat surrounded by bell peppers, onions, tomatoes, figs, eggplant, and other fruits from the Mediterranean vine.

Other research suggests that Mediterranean-style marinades used in Greek cooking may reduce the amount of a second type of carcinogen, heterocyclic amines (HCAs).

Marinating meats, even for just a few minutes before grilling or broiling, can reduce HCAs by 90 percent or more. There's no clearcut reason, but it may be the marinade sets up a barrier against heat, or that marinating draws out chemical precursors of carcinogens from the meat.

Apples: one a day keeps the oncologist away

Apples have been considered something special since the day one may have gotten Adam and Eve into trouble in the Garden of Eden. Nowadays only good things come from taking a bite from the once forbidden fruit.

Among the most commonly consumed popular fruits, apples are one of the richest sources of flavonoids like quercetin and phenolic acid, phytochemicals that are well-known to possess cancer-fighting qualities. The more you eat, the better they are for you. When researchers in Italy compared the apple consumption of more than 1,200 men, they found an apple a day can help keep prostate cancer at bay. Two a day offered even more protection.

To get the most nutrition out of eating an apple, don't throw away the peel. An apple's brilliant red skin is a sign of the presence of anthocyanins, nutrients baked into the skin by the sun and believed to be some of the most powerful cancer-fighting phytochemicals in the plant kingdom.

Apples are also a rich source of pectin, a fiber found to possess anti-cancer activities.

Berries: fighting cancer by the spoonful

Blueberries, strawberries, blackberries, raspberries — take your pick. You won't go wrong putting any one of them on your pro-prostate diet. Though tiny, berries are high-performing fruit, thanks to their rich assortment of cancer-fighting polyphenols.

There is a growing body of evidence that berries are powerful cancer fighters. Numerous test tube studies have found extracts from berries stop the growth and proliferation of human prostate cancer cells.

Rich, deep color is a sign of a berry's healthfulness. The color comes from anthocyanins, supercharged antioxidants enriched by the sun and found beneath the skin. Though all berries have beneficial health qualities, those that have been found to be associated with prostate health are:

- blackberries
- blueberries
- red raspberries
- black raspberries
- cranberries
- strawberries

Cabbages: meet the crucifer clan

When it comes to vegetables and preventing prostate disease, the operative word is cabbage. Several studies have found that men get special prostate protection when they eat heartily of cabbages and other vegetables that are in the large family known as crucifers.

Studies show that eating cabbages helps reduce the risk of cancer and BPH. It can also help reduce the lower urinary tract symptoms associated with BPH. One study involving more than 600 men and conducted by the National Cancer Institute found that men who ate three or more servings of cruciferous vegetables a week cut their risk of prostate cancer almost in half. A long-term analysis of the dietary habits of more than 32,000 men found that those who ate the most cruciferous vegetables had the lowest risk of BPH compared to men who ate the least. Cabbage eaters are also less likely to need surgery to correct the complaints of BPH.

The cabbage clan's prostate defense system is led by special substances called glucosinolates, which are converted into cancer-fighting isothiocyanates and sulforaphane, which produce the sulphur-like odor you detect when these vegetables are cooked. Researchers believe these substances promote prostate health by modulating the immune system and helping to regulate the balance of hormones in the prostate.

Even if you're not crazy about cabbage, you don't have to eat it every day to get its benefits. "Our findings provide evidence that two or more servings per month of cruciferous vegetables may reduce risk of prostate cancer," noted a study in the journal *Nutrition and Cancer*.

Broccoli reigns supreme. This stem of brilliant green buds is the most powerful of all cruciferous vegetables. Researchers at Mount Sinai Hospital in New York City found that men who ate the most cruciferous vegetables had the lowest incidence of prostate cancer, but men who ate the most broccoli had the lowest incidence of all.

Brussels sprouts are No. 2. These baby green cabbages are second only to broccoli as the richest source of glucosinolates. Eating Brussels sprouts is associated with a reduced risk of prostate cancer.

Cabbage offers something special. Cabbage — red, green, and savoy — contains a special substance called sinigrin, which has been found to offer its own brand of prostate protection.

Canola — a choice oil. Canola is a member of the cruciferous family — and a high-ranking one at that. You could call it the cabbage family's kissing cousin.

That's because canola oil is extracted from a special variety of seed originally bred in Canada from rapeseed. This variety bred out harmful components found in rapeseed oil, resulting in an oil that is especially healthy.

Canola, the mostly commonly used culinary oil in the world, is one of the richest sources of the prostate-protecting omega-3 fatty acid linolenic acid. Research shows that if men ate food made with canola oil in place of other vegetable oils, it would provide the optimal daily amount of omega-3s important to prostate health — and heart health would be greatly improved as well.

Cauliflower — one big bud. You'd think that this pale face couldn't hold a candle to its deep green brother broccoli, but that's not the case at all. Like broccoli, cauliflower's growth stops at the bud stage, which is why it has such a concentrated nutritional content — and such an interesting shape.

Collard greens — nutritional Southern charm. Animal studies show that this Southern staple contains 15 different cancer-tracking nutrients that go into action when the leaves are sliced or chewed. Collard greens also are a good source of other prostate-protecting nutrients, including beta carotene and vitamin E.

Hail for kale. This leafy green has a unique combination of more than 45 different cancer-fighting and prostate-protecting flavonoids and carotenoids.

Mustard greens cut the mustard. This bitter green is not to be ignored. It takes the number three spot in possessing prostate-protecting glucosinolates, meaning it's mighty healthy.

Watercress — more than a garnish. The nutritional strength of these greens defy their delicate nature. Experiments in the research laboratory at the University of Pittsburgh show watercress extracts can kill human prostate cancer cells in the test tube.

Chilies: a hot choice to put the brakes on aggressive cancer

This south-of-the-border staple is a hot sensation in the kitchen for the beloved spicy hot flavor it ignites in food, but it is a hot sensation in the research laboratory as well.

Chili's killer heat comes from an almost impossible-to-kill alkaloid called capsaicin, one of the most powerful antioxidants in the plant kingdom. Though eating chilies has an impressive roster of proven health benefits, research in the role they play in prostate health is only in its infancy. Preliminary studies, however, show it is so powerful it may be able to help stop even the most aggressive forms of prostate cancer. One study found that capsaicin from chilies stopped progression of disease in mice inoculated with prostate cancer cells that did not respond to testosterone-suppressing drugs.

Results like these are yet to be replicated in humans — except for the story of a man researchers believe slowed his rising PSA and the progression of his recurring prostate cancer by downing a spoonful of habanero chili sauce, made from one of the hottest peppers on Earth, a couple of times a week. The researchers describe what happened in a report in the *Canadian Urological Association Journal*.

The man, who was 66 at the time, had prostate cancer that had advanced to an aggressive stage after three years. Doctors started hormone replacement therapy to slow the disease, but the man stopped taking the drugs because he couldn't tolerate the side effects. As a result, his PSA rose to the point where it was doubling every four weeks — not a good sign to say the least. This is when he got into the chili sauce.

He began eating habanero chili sauce twice a week in April. By October, his PSA doubling time slowed from four weeks to seven months. When he stopped eating the sauce, his doctors reported, the doubling time got faster; when he resumed eating it, doubling time once again slowed down. "When the patient stopped capsaicin, a PSA rise or decrease in doubling time was consistently observed," noted the researchers. Though such a case is rare — virtually all studies have been conducted using supplements rather than food — it demonstrates that a healing effect is possible through eating chilies.

Capsaicin, noted the researchers, "may be useful in prevention, in slowing the growth of prostate cancer in patients on active surveillance, or in patients who have recurrent disease before the next line of definitive therapy."

The hot, hotter, and hottest

Chilies are the sole food source of capsaicin. In fact, capsaicin defines what a chili is all about. If a pepper has no heat, it has no capsaicin, and if it has no capsaicin, it's not a chili. The more capsaicin, the hotter the chili.

If you want to stoke your health fires, here are the hottest of the hot, ranked here by the chilies that contain the most capsaicin. (Warning: Some of these are so hot, they could be dangerous.)

1. Habanero

2. Scotch bonnet

3. Thai

4. Piquin

5. Cayenne

6. Tabasco

7. Manzano

8. Serrano

9. Chipotle

10. Jalapeno

(Also see *Capsaicin* on page 323.)

Citrus fruit: the best vitamin C solution

Citrus fruits high in vitamin C are high on the list of good-for-the-prostate fruits. Though only a limited number of studies have been conducted on citrus and prostate disease, they consistently show that the higher the intake of citrus fruit, the better the protection.

Most recently, a Japanese study that followed the eating habits of more than 42,000 men found that daily consumption of citrus fruit correlated to a reduced risk of all types of cancer.

Getting more citrus fruit in the diet also offers benefits to men with BPH. A study in the *American Journal of Clinical Nutrition* found that men with BPH who ate the most citrus fruit experienced fewer lower urinary tract complaints and were less likely to require invasive treatment than men who ate the least amount of citrus fruit. The fruits specifically cited for offering the most symptom relief were oranges and orange juice and grapefruit and grapefruit juice.

If you're looking to add more antioxidant vitamin C to your diet, your best bet is to eat more citrus fruits. There is little evidence that taking vitamin C supplements offers the same protection.

Extra C: no good news for LUTS

The Boston Area Community Health Survey questioned close to 1,500 men, ages 30 to 79, and found that those who took a high dose of supplemental vitamin C — at least 250 milligrams a day — were 83 percent more likely to have LUTS (lower urinary tract symptoms) than those who didn't take extra vitamin C. The researchers suspect the vitamin makes urine more acid which can lead to increased urgency. Try cutting back on supplemental vitamin C if you have LUTS and see if your urinary symptoms improve.

Cranberries: equal opportunity infection protection

The cranberry's reputation as a healer is spreading. Its well-known ability to prevent common urinary tract infections in women now has a counterpart in men as researchers have recently discovered. Cranberries can knock out painful symptoms of persistent, hard-to-treat chronic nonbacterial prostatitis.

Cranberry won its first round when it proved to be just as effective as the powerful antibiotic drug ciprofloxacin (Cipro) in preventing a flare-up of the disease in test animals. It moved to the winner's circle, however, when researchers found it could improve symptoms of the disease in men.

The experiment, published in the *British Journal of Nutrition*, involved using dried powdered cranberries as the only treatment in a small group of men with not only chronic nonbacterial prostatitis, but LUTS and elevated PSA levels, too. After six months of treatment, the men showed "statistically significant improvement" in all measurements of urination difficulties. Their PSA levels also dropped, a sign the infection was abating. By comparison, men in the same study who received no treatment experienced no symptom relief.

Cranberry gets its might from an arsenal of polyphenolic compounds, including anthocyanins found in the berry's skin. Studies in the United States and abroad are also investigating compounds in cranberry as a potential treatment for prostate cancer. Preliminary laboratory studies have found that it can stop the initiation and proliferation of human prostate tumors and prevent tumors from metastasizing — findings, noted researchers in *Nutrition and Cancer*, that "further establish the potential value of cranberry phytochemicals as possible agents against prostate cancer."

Fish: chewing the omega-3 fat

When was the last time you ate a meal that featured fish? If you ask that question to a man living in Japan, the answer most likely would be, "My last meal." The typical American male most likely would be clueless about the last time he ate fish.

Americans don't eat nearly enough fish for health, and men eat much less than women. The typical American male eats fish about once every two weeks, according to statistics, compared to Japanese men who eat it daily. So why does it matter? Because the Japanese diet, which is low in fatty red meat but high in fatty fish just might be the reason why Japanese men have one of the lowest incidences of prostate disease in the world. American men have nearly 20 times the rate of prostate cancer as Japanese men. It's a fact that has researchers debating: Is eating fish so healthy that it can reduce the risk of cancer? Or is the risk of prostate disease so low among Japanese men because they consume less red meat? Most likely, the answer is both. However, when it comes to prostate health, there is no underestimating the power of eating fish.

> American men have nearly 20 times the rate of prostate cancer as Japanese men.

The food trifecta

While rice is a staple of the Japanese diet, fish, soy, and green tea, three of the best foods to help prevent prostate enlargement and prostate cancer, are, in general, consumed daily.

A sea of evidence

Certain fish, such as the Japanese sushi favorites tuna and salmon, get their full-bodied flavor from a special kind of fat called omega-3 fatty acids that are essential to health but are not manufactured in the body. Researchers discovered the health-bestowing benefits of fatty fish more than 50 years ago when they began looking for the reason native North American Inuit enjoyed an unusually low rate of heart disease. It turned out to be their steady diet of fatty fish. Over the next several decades, researchers discovered omega-3 fatty acids help protect against many diseases and one of them is prostate cancer.

The evidence that eating fish benefits the prostate is as strong as the sea air in a summer wind. Numerous population studies have found that eating omega-3-rich fish a few times a week can help prevent prostate cancer, help stop it from spreading to other organs, and reduce your chances of dying from it. For example:

- One 20-year study of more than 20,000 men found that men who consumed fish five or more times a week had a 48 percent lower risk of dying from prostate cancer than men who consumed fish just once a week.

- A 12-year study involving nearly 48,000 men found that eating fish more than three times a week was associated with a reduced risk of getting metastatic prostate cancer.

- Researchers in San Francisco found that men who ate dark fish — defined as salmon, mackerel, or blue fish — three times a month had a 36 percent lower risk of prostate cancer than men who never ate dark fish. Men who ate the same amount of shellfish — shrimp, lobster, and oysters — showed a similar reduced risk for getting aggressive prostate cancer. In this study, even eating tuna noodle casserole, which contains unhealthy fats, was found to have a protective effect.

- In Sweden, where consumption of fatty fish is also high, researchers reported that eating just one serving of salmon a week reduced the risk of developing prostate cancer by 43 percent.

- An analysis of 12 major population studies on eating fish and prostate cancer found regular consumption of fish reduced the risk of dying from prostate disease on average by 63 percent.

Getting your omega-3s

If eating fish doesn't stir your appetite, try taking a fish oil supplement. It may offer your prostate the same protection as a healthy fish dinner. Read more about this supplement on page 297.

Fishing for better health

Unfortunately, there is an environmental problem with eating fish today that didn't exist in the days when Eskimos were fishing through ice holes in the frozen waters of Alaska — mercury that collects in the fatty flesh of fish, especially very large ocean-caught fish. All fish contain mercury, according to the U.S. Environmental Protection Agency (EPA), however large fatty finfish collect the most. Though most doctors and the EPA feel that the healthy benefits you garner from eating fish outweigh the risks, there are ways to minimize your exposure to mercury.

Limit your intake. Studies show you can get a prostate-protecting effect from eating as little as two or three servings a week of these fatty fish:

- herring
- salmon
- trout
- tuna
- sardines
- mackerel
- halibut

Go wild. Studies have found that farm-raised salmon contains much more mercury and environmental toxins than those caught in the open sea because contaminants collect in the farms' close breeding grounds. Supermarkets are the most popular outlets for farm-raised salmon — up to 90 percent of salmon filets sold in supermarkets and restaurants is farm-raised. Unfortunately, that implies the most available and least expensive salmon is the least desirable from the presence of environmental contaminants. But don't forget canned. Most canned salmon, identified on the label as caught wild in Alaskan waters and sold in the U.S, is the purest fish in the world, practically free of mercury. And it's inexpensive — what a benefit for your pocketbook.

Some markets try to pass off farm-raised fish as wild. If the fish is not marked "wild," specifically ask the fishmonger if the fish he is selling was farm-raised. A tip-off that you may not be getting wild salmon is price. Wild salmon can cost as much as $20 a pound. In the end, you'll know if you're eating wild salmon by its buttery taste.

To get the very best, dine out. The best and freshest fish are often put aside at the dock for restaurants. A survey of fine-dining establishments in the United States shows that 70 percent of the best eating fish goes to restaurants.

Grapes: prostate benefits in a bunch

Next time you're on the prowl for a prostate-healthy snack, make sure you pluck a few grapes — their skins are loaded with a natural compound called resveratrol. Plants produce it to protect themselves from stress, injury, fungal infection, and the sun's ultraviolet rays. It may also protect you and your prostate. Working as an antioxidant, experts believe resveratrol battles prostate cancer by slowing or stopping tumor growth.

Perhaps you've heard resveratrol mentioned as one of the healthy ingredients in red wine, but if you're not a drinker, grapes and resveratrol-laden grape juice can be healthy substitutes. You can also get this important substance from red-skinned peanuts, some berries, and one little-known native, southern U.S. grape — the muscadine. The scuppernong is a muscadine variety first known as the "big white grape," but is actually more green or bronze in color.

The muscadine, a tough-skinned but tasty grape often made into jams, preserves, and juice, generally has the highest amount of resveratrol of any grape. One serving of muscadine jam contains as much resveratrol as 4 ounces of red wine. Scientists have found that this modest fruit not only contains substantial amounts of resveratrol but is high in fiber and carbohydrates, and low in fat.

The amount of resveratrol in grapes varies widely, depending on the type of grape, region, soil, method of storage, and other factors. That can make it difficult to gauge just how much resveratrol you're getting. Read more about resveratrol supplements on page 296.

Green tea: the terminator

China has one of the lowest rates of prostate cancer in the world. The Chinese drink more green tea than any other nation in the world — 10 cups a day is considered normal! Research indicates there's a relationship between the two.

Further proof of green tea's protective nature is noted among Asian men who migrate to the United States and discontinue the ritual of drinking green tea: their incidence of prostate cancer goes up.

To say that green tea is healthy is an understatement. Research databases cite thousands of studies linking green tea to cancer prevention. Green tea's remarkable protective effect comes from catechins, antioxidants with well-known anti-cancer activity. Much of the credit, however, goes to a special brand of catechin called epigallocatechin gallate (EGCG), a particularly potent and active cell-protecting antioxidant that takes a shine to the prostate.

Population studies around the world have found that consuming green tea is associated with protection against all stages of prostate cancer. Research shows that green tea fights cancer at the cellular level by turning off the genes that initiate cancer growth. It can also follow cancerous cells that are starting to migrate and arrest them before they get the chance to escape. A large Japanese study involving nearly 50,000 men found that drinking five cups of green tea a day cut the risk of advanced prostate cancer in half.

When Chinese experts analyzed hundreds of studies spanning more than 40 years to ascertain green tea's true strength as a cancer fighter, they found the risk of prostate cancer went down as the frequency, duration, and quantity of green tea consumption went up. The researchers concluded that the greatest protection comes from drinking five or more cups a day, but even drinking one cup affords some defense.

Keeping good company

Green tea is the quintessential example of how foods, or more specifically the nutrients in foods, work better together than any food alone. Drinking green tea along with eating prostate-friendly foods gives your meal a nutritional boost.

One Asian study of 400 men found that eating lycopene-rich tomatoes and drinking green tea reduced the risk of prostate cancer by 86 percent. Drinking green tea also offered extra prostate protection to Japanese men who enjoyed eating vitamin C-rich citrus fruits followed by green tea.

Getting the most from your tea

Green tea has a shelf life that seemingly goes on forever. Unfortunately, EGCG does not. When researchers stored green tea under prime conditions — in a cool, dark place — they found that the tea lost a little of its prostate-protecting power as each week went by. By six months it lost more than a quarter of its potency. So buy green tea according to your drinking habits. Since you most likely won't know how long the tea has been sitting on a store's shelf, buy enough to last no more than a month or two.

(Also see *Green Tea Extract* on page 289.)

Licorice: candy for the prostate

There is "licorice," the kind of candy kids love in an infinite number of color flavors, and there is real licorice, with a full-bodied flavor that makes most kids wrinkle their noses. Most licorice candies contain no real licorice, just a flavoring often made from the herb anise. You can, however, find real licorice in specialty food stores.

If you have an enlarged prostate, it's worth developing a taste for true licorice. It contains compounds that prevent the conversion of the male hormone testosterone to dihydrotestosterone, the active form believed to fuel the prostate growth that results in BPH.

The side effects, however, may not be worth it. Eating a lot of real licorice over an extended period of time can produce side effects, such as headaches and fatigue. In addition, because real licorice contains glycyrrhizic acid, it can cause your body to retain salt and fluids, and lose potassium — a double whammy that raises blood pressure.

Mustard and mustard seeds: a healthy topping

Bright yellow mustard may be as American as a ballpark frank, but we're considered latecomers when it comes to appreciating the value of mustard seeds — as a condiment, as a spice, and as a healing agent.

Mustard seeds come from mustard greens, though not the same mustard greens we put in soups and salads. That puts mustard seeds in the cabbage family, making them a cruciferous spice.

Though very small, there is a lot of might in a tablespoon of mustard seeds. When mustard seeds are exposed to cold water, they release an enzyme called myrosinase that activates sulphur-like compounds called glucosinolates, the same substance that makes cruciferous vegetables potent cancer fighters. It is also the substance that gives mustard its distinctive bite.

Though no studies have been conducted on mustard seeds and prostate cancer protection, hundreds of studies have found that glucosinolates help fight several types of cancer, including prostate cancer.

And researchers are investigating mustard seeds and mustard powder as protective agents against another prostate problem: BPH. Preliminary research in China found that glucosinolates found in mustard seeds stopped the growth of enlarging prostates in test animals.

So take advantage of mustard as a condiment. Both the powder and seeds are used to make prepared mustards, which come in a wide range of temperatures, from mild to tongue-scorching, and an infinite number of flavorings.

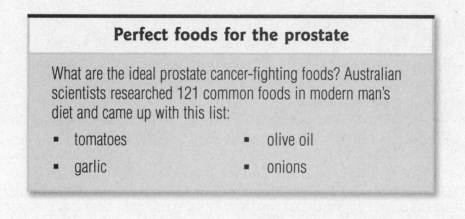

Perfect foods for the prostate

What are the ideal prostate cancer-fighting foods? Australian scientists researched 121 common foods in modern man's diet and came up with this list:

- tomatoes
- garlic
- olive oil
- onions

Olive oil: pouring with good health

The Mediterranean diet is high in fat. Nearly 40 percent of the daily calories of people who live in Greece and the island of Crete comes from fat. That's right up there with American fat consumption. The difference is that Americans eat an abundance of saturated fat — the kind found in butter, red meat, and fast food — while virtually all the fat consumed by Greeks comes in the form of olive oil. And that makes a big fat difference between what is so bad about the Western style of eating and what's so good about the way Greeks eat.

Olive oil is proof perfect that it isn't fat, but the type of fat, that is important when it comes to good health — and a healthy prostate. When researchers in Greece examined the Mediterranean diet and its affect on health, they concluded that the incidence of prostate cancer in the United States would drop 10 percent if American men replaced butter with olive oil.

Olive oil is rich in one of the "good fats," oleic acid, a type of monounsaturated fatty acid. But it also contains a smaller amount of polyunsaturated fat and natural antioxidants called polyphenols shown to have a host of beneficial effects. Out of all the foods on the Mediterranean diet, olive oil is considered by many to be the best of the best. Hundreds of studies that have examined the Mediterranean diet give olive oil the lion's share of the credit for Greece's low rate of heart disease and certain types of cancer, including prostate cancer.

Among the authors of these studies are researchers from the Harvard School of Public Health and the University of Athens Medical School. "Different countries and regions in the Mediterranean basin have their own dietary traditions, but in all of them olive oil occupies a central position," they commented in a joint review on cancer and Mediterranean dietary traditions. "From a health point of view, olive oil is important, not only because it has in itself beneficial properties, but also because it facilitates the consumption of large quantities of vegetables and legumes in the form of raw salads and cooked foods."

Indeed. Greeks love olive oil and pour it on at every meal. It is so central to their style of eating that a bottle of olive oil sits on the dining table in homes and restaurants just like a bottle of ketchup in a hamburger haven in the United States.

Extra virgin: the symbol of quality

Small boutique olive groves in Greece are reputed to produce the world's best, and healthiest, olive oil — cloudy, thick, and deep golden green, extra virgin oil.

To be extra virgin, the oil must be extracted from the fruit without altering the oil and without any treatment other than washing, decanting, and filtration. Extra virgin oil comes from the first pressing and ranges from golden yellow to almost bright green in color. The greener the oil, the better the quality, and the higher its polyphenol content. Extra virgin olive oil contains 30 different polyphenols, each with its own demonstrated anti-cancer qualities. The most important are squalene, lignans, and tyrosol — all nutrients associated with a reduced risk of prostate cancer.

The quality of olive oil is dependent on its acid content. The more refining, or filtering, the oil goes through, the higher the acid level. The greener the oil, the less acid it contains. To be labeled extra virgin, the acid content cannot be more than 1 percent. Look for the designation *extra nonfiltre* on the label.

Olive oil is somewhat temperamental and can lose its health-promoting polyphenol content if it's exposed to heat or sunlight or if it is stored too long. Studies show polyphenol content starts to diminish after about three months. By six months, it can lose as much as 40 percent of its nutritive value. So buy olive oil in a size that fits your typical usage.

Pomegranate juice and seeds: mega-trendy protection

Considering a lot of people in the United States never even heard of pomegranate a decade or so ago, it has created quite a stir — and not just in the martini pitcher.

Pomegranate juice became a health drink — and pomegranate martinis followed soon after — back in the '90s when studies started to emerge linking it to heart and prostate health. Today, pomegranate seeds — the glistening ruby red sac found when you break open the inedible fruit — and its juice are so trendy you can find them flavoring everything from mashed potatoes to specialty cocktails.

Pomegranate owes its nutritional riches to its unique chemistry of cancer-fighting antioxidants. While there are many foods abundant in polyphenols, pomegranate is believed to be the only one that is a source of all varieties of polyphenols — tannins, flavonoids, anthocyanins, and the most intriguing, ellagic acid. Researchers believe these nutrients work synergistically to make pomegranate a super-healthy food. Four different testing methods found that pomegranate seed extracts and juice have an antioxidant arsenal two to three times more powerful than any other food. And one of the beneficiaries is the prostate.

Drinking pomegranate juice is proving to be a tasty preventive strategy for men on active surveillance for prostate cancer and men who have been treated for the disease. Studies show that drinking a glass of pomegranate juice a day can help bring down elevated PSA levels.

In one study, researchers at UCLA gave 8 ounces of pomegranate juice a day to men with rising PSAs, despite having been treated for prostate cancer by either a radical prostatectomy or radiation. At the time of the experiment, the men's average PSA doubling time — for example, the time it takes PSA to rise from a 4 to an 8 — was 15 months. After the treatment, doubling time was more than four years! The researchers also found pomegranate juice therapy helped decrease the growth of cancer cells by 12 percent and induced a 17 percent increase in cancer cell death.

"There are limited treatment options for prostate cancer patients who have undergone primary therapy such as radical prostatectomy but have progressive elevation of their PSA," commented David Heber, M.D., one of the study researchers, in the journal *Cancer Letters*. "Our data on pomegranate juice given daily for two years to 40 prostate cancer patients with rising PSA provides a nontoxic option for prevention or delay of prostate carcinogenesis. It is remarkable that 85 percent of patients responded to pomegranate juice in this study."

Getting all juiced up

Pomegranate is a seasonal fruit available from October through January. This is the only time you can crack open the round fruit and enjoy its fresh juicy seeds. Pomegranate juice, however, is available year-round. Be forewarned, pomegranate juice is expensive. It is also high-calorie. An 8-ounce glass is around 150 calories.

(Also see *Ellagic Acid* on page 316.)

Pomegranate as a spice

In India, where rates of prostate problems are the lowest, pomegranate has been popular for centuries — but as a spice, not a juice. People in India dry the seeds as a spice called anardana, which is used to flavor curries, chutneys, pakoras (sweet dried snacks), and parathas (flat breads).

Pumpkin seeds: relief from the symptoms of BPH

The next time your kids are carving out a pumpkin for their Halloween jack o' lantern, ask them to save you the seeds. Pumpkin seeds are packed with special nutrients that have been well-known for decades as a tasty way to help control an enlarged prostate. In fact, many men in southern Europe eat a handful a day as a way to prevent prostate trouble.

Pumpkin seeds contain prostate-protecting compounds rarely found together in one edible substance. They are rich in antioxidant phenols, phytosterols, omega-3 fatty acids, zinc, and antioxidant vitamin E. They are also a good source of protein. Researchers speculate this unique nutritional profile is what makes pumpkin seeds so effective at relieving the lower urinary tract symptoms that plague men with BPH. It appears pumpkin seeds work in the same fashion as the BPH prescription medication alpha blockers — by preventing testosterone from manufacturing dihydrotestosterone, which acts like fuel for prostate growth.

Several studies have found that eating pumpkin seeds or taking a pumpkin seed extract brought relief to men with moderate to severe urinary tract troubles caused by an enlarged prostate.

In one study conducted in Korea, 47 men with BPH were treated with 320 milligrams of pumpkin seed extract twice a day for a year. After three months, improvement was seen in all physical symptoms. In comparison to men who took a placebo and found no relief, the men who took the pumpkin extract experienced a 58 percent overall improvement in the International Prostate Symptom Score, which rates the quality of life for men with BPH. The researchers found the extract to be clinically safe and suggested it may be "an effective alternative treatment for BPH."

In another study from Sweden, researchers gave pumpkin seed extract twice a day to men with BPH so severe they needed surgery. Not only did the treatment help them avoid surgery, the men found significant relief from all symptoms after three months of treatment.

Pumpkin seeds have an added advantage that benefits men with BPH. They act as a natural diuretic, which helps encourage urine flow. Men who took pumpkin seed extract found it also decreased the urgency and frequency of nighttime urination.

The downside to eating pumpkin seeds is that lowering the active form of testosterone in your body has side effects — such as reduced energy and libido, and erectile dysfunction.

Pumpkin seeds are a tasty snack you can eat out of hand. You can also sprinkle them on salads and mix them in yogurt.

Raisins: more than a trace of protection

Boron isn't exactly a household word, even among nutritional scientists. In fact, boron traditionally had been dismissed as biologically irrelevant until researchers started to notice that men with the lowest risk of prostate cancer had high levels of boron in their blood.

It is a trace mineral that the body requires only in miniscule amounts. Our need for it is so minute, in fact, that there isn't even a daily value (DV) for it, though it is included in many multiple vitamin formulations.

Boron is found in drinking water and in small amounts in a variety of fruits, vegetables, nuts, and seeds, although the amount in a food can vary according to the quality of soil. Raisins are the chief source, containing twice as much as any other food. In addition to raisins, boron is most abundant in these foods:

- almonds
- apples
- avocados
- hazelnuts
- peanut butter
- pears
- prunes

One UCLA study involving several thousand men found that those who consumed at least 1.8 milligrams of boron a day had less than a third of the risk of developing prostate cancer as men who consumed half as much boron.

"Our research suggests higher boron levels lower the risk of prostate cancer by reducing cancer cell signaling and storage," commented the researchers.

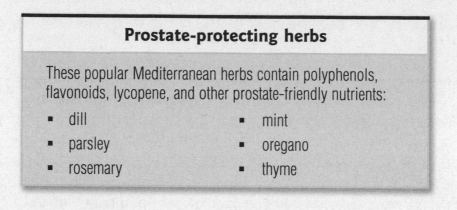

Prostate-protecting herbs

These popular Mediterranean herbs contain polyphenols, flavonoids, lycopene, and other prostate-friendly nutrients:

- dill
- parsley
- rosemary
- mint
- oregano
- thyme

Rosemary: keep it by the grill

Walk along the sandy scrublands of the Mediterranean Sea and you'll likely get a whiff of the pine-like scent of rosemary growing wild among the dunes.

Rosemary is one of the most popular and versatile herbs associated with Mediterranean cuisine. The Greeks are particularly fond of it and use it in just about everything. They also bundle it and throw it on the barbecue so its seductive scent penetrates grilled fish, meats, and vegetables — a practice that helps protect the prostate in a very special way.

The prostate is sensitive to heterocyclic amines (HCAs), carcinogens that build up in meats and fish that are grilled or fried at high temperatures. Rosemary, however, helps neutralize HCAs. Researchers at Kansas State University consistently have found that sprinkling foods with rosemary prior to grilling significantly reduced the buildup of these harmful chemicals.

For its small size, rosemary is an antioxidant powerhouse, which comes from a unique blend of cancer-fighting substances, including its namesake rosmarinic acid. When scientists in Turkey extracted these special compounds from rosemary leaves and put them in a petri dish with cancer cells from six different organs, including the prostate, they found it stopped the growth of all of them. Rosemary, concluded the researchers, "is a potential candidate to be included in the anti-cancer diet."

Soy: thumbs up for Asian style

Unless you're a vegetarian, you probably aren't all that tuned in to soy. In fact, if it weren't for the popularity of the soybean snack edamame, soy wouldn't make most men's most-wanted list. But you might want to reconsider. People in Japan and China, who eat soy foods daily, also have one of the lowest rates of prostate cancer in the world.

Hundreds of studies have found that soy is one of the diet's major allies in the battle against prostate cancer. For example:

- An analysis of eight major studies concluded that there is a link between high consumption of soy foods and a low incidence of prostate cancer. Tofu, noted researchers in the journal *Nutrition and Cancer*, stood out as one of the strongest anti-prostate cancer foods.

- In China, researchers found that a high intake of tofu, soymilk, and fermented soybeans was proportionate to the low rate of prostate cancer.

- Studies in men with prostate cancer have found that eating soy foods decreased their risk of the disease spreading to other organs and lowered their risk of dying from the disease.

Soy's prostate protection comes from its abundance of isoflavones, specifically genistein and daidzein. Soy is also rich in phytoestrogens that, as their name implies, are akin to the female hormone estrogen. Researchers believe that isoflavones in soy foods help protect the balance of hormones in the prostate and help prevent testosterone from manufacturing dihydrotesterone (DHT), which is implicated in causing both prostate cancer and BPH. One study found that three months of daily supplementation with soy isoflavones significantly decreased the level of circulating DHT in healthy Japanese men.

Unfortunately, consuming soy means that the undesirable effects of lowering DHT on libido and energy are also accentuated. In addition, a major study of Hawaiian men of Japanese descent showed that those who ate the most soy had greatly elevated rates of dementia, possibly linked to the almost unique isoflavones found in soy.

Seeking soy in all the right places

To get a prostate-protecting effect from soy, experts recommend getting a minimum of three or four servings of soy products a week.

Common soy foods include:

- tofu, a vegetarian meat and protein substitute that is sold in blocks

- tempeh, which is similar to tofu but firmer

- edamame, cooked soybeans

- miso, a fermented bean paste that forms the basis of miso soup as well as other Japanese dishes

- natto, fermented soybeans

- soy sauces, including shoyu, tamari, and teriyaki

- soymilk, which is vegetable-based and lactose-free

- soy cheese, which is made from soymilk

- soy ice cream and soy yogurt

- soybean oil, which can be used as a substitute for other oils in cooking

(Also see *Genistein* on page 319.)

Getting all steamed up!

When it comes to retaining the nutrients in cooked vegetables, water is enemy No. 1, according to research conducted in Spain.

In the experiment, the researchers cooked 20 top antioxidant-rich vegetables by different cooking methods to find out which retained the most nutrients. Steaming and microwaving retained the most nutrients. Boiling was the worst, causing an overall 50 percent nutrition loss.

Spinach: the king of greens

It's no secret that spinach is good for you when you have a famous cartoon character flexing his biceps every time he throws a can of the greens down his throat. It's a good bet that all that spinach has also given Popeye a strong and healthy prostate.

The deep green color of spinach leaves is the key sign of spinach's uniquely rich and active profile of cancer-fighting flavonoids. One study of more than 30,000 men found that eating spinach was more protective than any other vegetable except broccoli in lowering the risk of prostate cancer.

Though few studies have been conducted on spinach versus prostate cancer, the few controlled studies conducted to date have produced results nothing short of astounding. They found spinach wilts cancer at the cellular level and can even knock back the Brutus of prostate cancer — the kind that kills. One study found that the risk of developing aggressive treatment-resistant prostate cancer was lowest in men with the highest intake of spinach. And what would that intake be? Just two servings a week.

Spinach is quite hardy and retains much of its cancer-scavenging activity during cooking. Wilting it briefly in a sauté pan and using it in a stir-fry actually increases its nutritional power.

The Okinawa Diet

Diet has been cited as the reason for the low incidence of prostate disease on the Japanese island of Okinawa, where prostate cancer is about 80 percent less common than in North America. These are the foods that have been given the credit:

- colorful fruits and vegetables, including watermelons, yams, guavas, grapefruit, and tomatoes
- soy foods
- fish
- green tea

Tomatoes: now we're cookin'!

When it comes to protecting your prostate, a man can't go wrong eating anything with cooked tomatoes in it or on top. Pizza, pasta, ketchup, tomato paste, and tomato juice make the good-for-you list due to a very special secret ingredient — lycopene. Throw some olive oil on top and you get a gold star.

Of all the foods known to boost prostate health, the tomato and all its ancillary products are near the top.

Tomatoes — any variety from fresh plum and beefsteak to ketchup and canned spaghetti sauce — are rich in prostate-protecting lycopene, a particularly powerful member of a family of cancer-fighting phyto-chemicals known as carotenoids. More than 85 percent of lycopene that naturally exists is found in the tomato.

You'd think eating for prostate health couldn't get any better, but it does. Unlike other foods that lose some of their nutritional power when cooked, lycopene levels dramatically rise when tomatoes get cooked into pasta sauce, bottled as ketchup, or spread as a sauce over pizza dough. There is more lycopene in tomato sauce than a fresh tomato and more lycopene in tomato paste than tomato sauce.

Because of its chemical structure, lycopene expands when cooked in olive oil, making pasta and pizza sauces nutritionally potent. It all means that you can feel right at home in a pizza parlor. Here are just a few of the reasons why.

> ■ When researchers combined the findings of 21 studies on tomatoes and prostate cancer, they found that men who ate the most raw tomatoes had an 11 percent lower risk of prostate cancer than men who ate the least amount of raw tomatoes. Men who ate the most cooked tomatoes had a 19 percent reduced risk.

- A large dietary study involving more than 50,000 male health professionals found that consuming two to four servings of tomato sauce a week was associated with a 35 percent reduced risk of getting prostate cancer and a 50 percent reduced risk of getting an aggressive form of the disease.

- PSA levels dropped nearly 11 percent in men with BPH who ate meals containing 2 ounces of tomato paste every day for 10 weeks, according to Brazilian researchers.

- In one study, doctors in Chicago had a small group of men eat pasta with tomato sauce every day for three weeks prior to having surgery for prostate cancer. When pathologists analyzed the cancerous areas in their prostates after surgery, they found that many of the cancerous cells that were active at biopsy were dead. This was not the case in a similar group of men who avoided eating tomato products prior to surgery.

- One large-scale study looked at the consumption of 46 fruits and vegetables associated with a lower risk of prostate cancer. They found that eating tomato sauce, tomato juice, or pizza more than 10 times a week was associated with the lowest risk of prostate cancer.

Pass the pizza, please

Dig in! It's not No. 1, but pizza came in as the No. 3 richest source of prostate-protecting lycopene in a study by researchers at the Harvard School of Public Health. Beating it as the top lycopene-rich foods were ketchup followed by tomato juice!

These also happen to be the top three tomato-based favorites of American men. At least we're doing something right!

The whole tomato advantage

Though there's a mountain of research that says tomatoes are good for your prostate, some studies show they have no effect on prostate health at all. This is because scientists were only looking at lycopene, say researchers at Ohio State University, and lycopene works best in the company of other nutrients. To prove the point, the researchers put tomatoes head-to-head with broccoli, another famous pro-prostate vegetable.

For the experiment, the researchers fed powdered extracts of the two vegetables to test rats three different ways. One group was fed a diet containing 10 percent broccoli, another got 10 percent tomato, and the third received a diet consisting of 5 percent broccoli and 5 percent tomato. In human terms, this translates to four cups of broccoli and a cup of tomato sauce a day. The researchers also gave a fourth and fifth team supplemental lycopene in two different dosages. A month into the diet, the researchers injected the rats with prostate tumors. Nearly two years later, the scientists examined the rats for tumor growth.

All five combinations reduced tumor size, but the tomatoes and broccoli team had the best results — a 52 percent shrinkage. Broccoli alone reduced tumor size by 42 percent and the tomatoes alone reduced it 34 percent. The largest dosage of lycopene resulted in an 18 percent reduction and the smaller dosage reduced tumor size by 7 percent.

"Our findings strongly suggest that risks of poor dietary habits cannot be reversed simply by taking a pill," commented Steven Clinton, one of the Ohio State researchers. "If we want the health benefits of tomatoes, we should eat tomatoes or tomato products and not rely on lycopene supplements alone."

(Also see *Lycopene* on page 293.)

An ideal marriage

A study out of Athens, Greece suggested that the rate of prostate cancer would go down 40 percent if men ate more tomatoes and olive oil and avoided dairy products.

Walnuts: snacking on vitamin E

When searching for a healthy snack for prostate health, you can't do better than a handful of walnuts. This staple of the traditional Cretan diet headlines a stellar list of pro-prostate nutrients: monounsaturated fat, omega-3 fatty acids, ellagic acid, and vitamin E.

Several studies have found that eating a handful of walnuts a day has a positive effect on prostate health, and a great deal of the credit goes to vitamin E. Walnuts contain an unusually high level of a special kind of vitamin E called gamma-tocopherol, which is not the kind always found in dietary supplements.

When researchers from Pennsylvania State University asked a group of men with prostate cancer to add 2.5 ounces of walnuts to their typical diet for two months, they found that it improved biomarkers for their cancer as well as heart disease. Even though the walnuts added 463 calories to their daily diet, the men didn't gain any weight because they ate the walnuts as a substitute for other saturated fat in their diets.

Walnuts, said the researchers, have "significant benefits for both vascular and prostate health."

All tree nuts have vitamin E and many nutritionists believe similar benefits can be derived from eating any of them. They recommend an ounce a day.

The tree of health

These nuts all contain prostate-healthy vitamin E:

- Brazil nuts
- cashews
- hazelnuts
- macadamia nuts
- pecans
- pine nuts
- pistachios

Whole grains: hearty options for a healthy prostate

Almost every meal in the traditional Cretan diet is accompanied by large quantities of whole-grain bread, eaten just plain or dipped in a little extra virgin olive oil. Researchers believe it's a tradition central to good prostate health.

Population studies around the world show that eating a diet rich in whole grains, as well as fruits and vegetables, reduces the risk of many types of cancer, including prostate cancer. For example, in India, where whole grains constitute 60 to 70 percent of the diet, men enjoy the lowest rate of prostate cancer in the world.

Whole grains are important to prostate health for two reasons, according to researchers. They help maintain hormone balance and they prevent excess levels of insulin in the bloodstream, both of which are important in preventing prostate cancer and BPH.

Eating whole grains, however, is even more important to men who already have prostate cancer, according to some studies. In one pilot study, researchers in California recruited men who were experiencing rising PSA after having surgery or radiation therapy for prostate cancer. The rising PSA was a sign that the cancer was returning. The men were asked to add more whole grains and vegetables to their diets as a means to control the cancer. After three months, their median consumption of whole grains went from less than two servings a day to seven. They increased their vegetable intake from three to five servings daily. As their diet improved, the researchers noticed the rate at which their PSAs were rising began to slow down. When they went off the diet, PSA started to rise at a faster rate.

You'll get the best protection from not just eating more whole grains, but eliminating all refined grains from your diet.

Don't forget your water

A healthy diet includes plenty of water, and keeping you hydrated is only one of the reasons.

Water is a natural detoxifier. It helps your liver rid your body of potentially harmful carcinogens by flushing them out of your system. Alternative doctors recommend drinking at least eight to 10 glasses of water a day as a natural body purifier.

If you find it hard to guzzle that much water, remember you can keep your body hydrated by eating soup or water-filled produce — like grapefruit, watermelon, pineapple, or cucumbers — and by drinking juice, milk, or herbal tea.

Watch your glycemic index

Cancer cells are greedy and need energy to grow — energy you feed them through the foods in your diet. Blood sugar, or glucose, makes a convenient feeding trough for cancer cells. However, it is not blood sugar per se that is suspected of fueling prostate cancer but the insulin that is released when blood sugar rises.

Recent research suggests that there may be a connection between high levels of circulating insulin and the risk of prostate cancer. One study conducted by the National Cancer Institute found that men with the highest blood levels of insulin had a prostate cancer risk eight-and-a-half times greater than men with the lowest levels of insulin. One finding that supports this theory is the fact that men with diabetes, a disease of insulin deficiency, have a low incidence of prostate cancer.

Whenever you eat, glucose is released into the blood as part of the digestive process. Glucose triggers the release of insulin, a hormone that regulates carbohydrate and fat metabolism. As blood sugar rises, insulin release accelerates. Certain foods will cause glucose to rise slow and steady, releasing a slow and steady stream of insulin. These are called low-glycemic foods. Other foods, however, cause a rapid rise in glucose, which spurs a rapid release of insulin to chase it away.

> Men with the highest blood levels of insulin had a prostate cancer risk eight-and-a-half times greater than men with the lowest levels of insulin.

The best way to control the release of excess insulin is to eat foods that raise blood sugar slowly, just as people with diabetes are supposed to do. Nutritionists have "followed" the rate at which individual foods respond to glucose and insulin release and have attributed a number to them based on a standard called the glycemic index. The foods are ranked on a scale from 0 to 100, with 55 being the number that divides the good from the bad, meaning your target is foods that fall in the range from 0 to 54. For example, whole grains are low-glycemic foods and refined grains are generally high-glycemic foods. Rye bread has a glycemic index of 50 compared to a French baguette, which has a glycemic index of 95. Potatoes come in at 76.

The glycemic index and a complete list of foods are available on numerous sites on the Internet. Just Google "glycemic index."

The ideal prostate-protecting plate du jour

The picture perfect, prostate-protecting menu would look something like this:

Breakfast

   Orange juice

   Hot oatmeal sprinkled with assorted berries

   Two slices of whole-grain bread

Snack

   Glass of pomegranate juice

   Apple

Lunch

   Tomato soup

   Grilled curried chicken breast with grilled red onions and bean sprouts on five-grain bread

   Peppered cabbage

   A small salad of greens with balsamic vinaigrette

   Sliced mango and papaya with low-fat Greek yogurt

   Iced green tea

Snack

   Edamame

Dinner

   Whole-wheat pasta with red sauce

   Salmon or tuna sautéed in olive oil and garlic and sprinkled with mustard dill sauce

   Large salad of greens with red onion, tomatoes, walnuts, and cured olives, dressed with extra virgin olive oil, balsamic vinegar, and oregano

   Steamed broccoli

   Stewed tomatoes

   Glass of red grape juice

Supplemental insurance: nutritional protection

The lure is everywhere: The only supplement you'll ever need to protect your prostate ... Your best solution for the symptoms of an enlarged prostate ... The all-in-one formula that's a man's best friend.

The shelves of health food stores and pharmacies are bulging with a mind-boggling number of products promising to come to the rescue of your ailing prostate. Sifting through them and separating the facts from the hype can be maddening. Unfortunately, the Federal Drug Administration (FDA) isn't much help. It has opted to take a hands-off attitude when it comes to regulating the supplement industry.

So where does this leave you? Most likely in the same boat as most men — confused. Can a capsule offer the same nutritional value found in food? How do supplements work? Which supplements have been proven to be prostate-friendly and which are no better than snake oil? Most important, which supplement or supplements, if any, are right for you?

Researchers are investigating dozens of nutrients and herbs for their potential to help prevent and treat prostate disease. Many possess known anti-cancer qualities that may protect the prostate against cancer. Others are being tested as a treatment for the disease. Some have the potential to ease the bothersome lower urinary tract symptoms of benign prostatic hyperplasia (BPH) or shrink an enlarged prostate. Nothing, however, has been proven to be a cure.

Common-sense rules

The idea that taking a supplement or even a group of supplements will provide all the nutrition you need to protect your prostate is simplistic.

Supplements are no substitute for eating healthy foods that may contain the same nutrient. Isolating a potentially beneficial substance from food generally is less effective than eating the whole food that contains the substance.

For general prostate health and maintenance, specialists say that you should only take nutritional supplements in addition to, and not in lieu of, a healthy diet. Your best protection comes from following an overall healthy lifestyle, as outlined in Chapter 9.

First, some caveats

When it comes to keeping your prostate healthy, stoking your diet with nutritional supplements might be a good idea, especially if your diet is, shall we say, less than ideal. Any nutritionist or doctor, however, will tell you that a supplement is no substitute for a good diet or a panacea for your prostate problem. If you are being treated for prostate disease, or any other disease, do not take any supplements without discussing it with your doctor first. Also, never substitute a supplement for any prostate medication you may be taking. In addition, be mindful of these other caveats.

Ask your doctor. Make sure to ask your primary care physician and your urologist, if you're seeing one, about all the supplements you plan to take and in what amounts. This is particularly important if you are currently on active surveillance for prostate cancer or are being treated for a prostate condition. Dietary supplements can also interfere with the outcome of surgery. Ask your doctor again about taking them before surgery.

More is not better. Just because it is natural does not mean it is safe. Many supplements, including vitamins and minerals, can be toxic in high amounts. Do not exceed a recommended dosage.

Be careful of mixing supplements with medication. Some supplements can make certain medications ineffective or too effective — another reason to make the decision to supplement in consultation with your doctor.

Pay attention to side effects. Like medications, supplements have the potential for side effects, though they may be mild and rare. Anyone, however, can experience an allergic reaction, such as hives, itching, or difficulty breathing. If you experience any of these symptoms, seek immediate medical attention.

Keep your supplements in a safe place. This means out of reach of children and pets.

This chapter highlights the substances scientists are researching for clues that may lead to the prevention and treatment of prostate disease. They include vitamins, minerals, phytochemicals, and herbs, ranging from the tried-and-true to the speculative and controversial. Virtually all of them are sold as supplements or packaged in formulas claiming to promote prostate health.

To help you sort through the maze of information and misinformation out there on these substances, they are grouped according to the strength of the research that currently exists.

Group 1

These supplements are supported by years of research and human studies. They show the most promise for prostate health.

Aspirin: thinning your cancer risk

Aspirin isn't exactly a supplement, but for decades doctors have been treating it like one for heart health. It's possible that some day soon doctors will be just as likely to recommend it for the prostate.

There is now ample proof that taking an aspirin a day helps lower the risk of prostate cancer. It also holds significant promise of greatly increasing survival for men with high-risk disease.

Numerous studies, including one involving 29,000 men, found that taking a daily aspirin or other nonsteroidal anti-inflammatory drug (NSAID) reduced the risk of prostate cancer by an average of 14 percent. In men who reported taking two or more NSAIDs a day, the reduced risk was even better — 21 percent. And an analysis of 24 studies involving 24,230 men by researchers at the University of Arizona in Tucson concluded that a daily NSAID is "suggestive of reduced risk" of prostate cancer.

A study involving more than 5,000 men undergoing either surgery or radiation therapy for prostate cancer found that men who took a daily aspirin prior to treatment had a 50 percent reduced risk of the cancer returning than men who didn't take aspirin. This statistic included men in the most advanced stage of the disease.

"Evidence has shown that anticoagulants may interfere with cancer growth and spread," said Kevin Choe, M.D., Ph.D., of the University of Texas Southwestern Medical School in Dallas, Texas, where the study took place.

Scientists believe aspirin works by blocking the effects of COX enzymes, proteins involved in inflammation that are often found to be high in men with prostate cancer. In fact, taking any anti-clotting drug is proving to be protective against prostate cancer.

In a study at the University of Chicago, researchers examined the effect of taking the anti-clotting medications Coumadin and Plavix, as well as aspirin, in 662 men undergoing radiation treatment for prostate cancer. Of the total, 196 were taking aspirin, 58 were taking Coumadin, and 24 were taking Plavix. The rest of the men weren't taking any anti-clotting medications.

Four years after treatment, cancer recurred in only 9 percent of the men taking the medication compared to 22 percent in the men who didn't take any medication. Here, too, the benefit was most pronounced in men with high-risk aggressive cancer. In the high-risk group, cancer recurred in 18 percent of men on anticoagulants compared to 42 percent of men not taking the drugs.

Researchers caution men with prostate cancer to not take anticoagulants without the consent of their oncologist, as the medications carry their own risk, including internal bleeding.

Talk to your doctor about the correct aspirin dosage for you. It's generally safer than other nonsteroidal anti-inflammatories (NSAIDs), with fewer side effects and more overall positive health benefits than negatives.

Vitamin D: don't forget the sunshine vitamin

The United States is in the midst of a nutritional crisis: The majority of Americans are deficient in vitamin D, the so-called sunshine vitamin.

Vitamin D is essential to health, much more so than doctors and researchers ever realized. At one time, a vitamin D deficiency was only associated with rickets in children and bone loss in adults, but studies during the last several years have discovered that vitamin D is protective against a wide variety of diseases. One of them may be prostate cancer. The Prostate Cancer Prevention Trial involving nearly 5,000 men concluded that vitamin D has a protective effect against prostate disease.

"There is overwhelming scientific evidence that increased exposure to sunlight, which increases vitamin D3 synthesis and a person's vitamin D status, can influence the risk for an outcome of many deadly cancers," said Michael F. Holick, M.D., Ph.D., a vitamin D expert and researcher at Boston University Medical Center in Boston. "It is estimated that there is a 30 to 50 percent reduction in risk for developing colorectal, breast, and prostate cancer by either increasing vitamin D intake to 1,000 IU a day or increasing sun exposure." Studies show that as exposure to ultraviolet light increases, mortality from prostate cancer decreases.

In a pilot study of men who got recurrent prostate cancer after treatment with surgery or radiation, researchers at Stanford University School of Medicine found that therapeutic dosages of vitamin D "significantly decreased" the rate of rising PSA in six out of seven men.

The high rate of vitamin D deficiency is attributed primarily to insufficient outdoor activity and the overzealous use of sunscreen. While overexposure to sunlight may increase the incidence of skin cancer, you must weigh this downside against the great overall benefit of vitamin D.

Those most at risk are believed to be people who live in the northeast and those with a lot of melanin in the skin, a pigment that protects against ultraviolet rays of the sun, such as black men. In fact, Dr. Holick believes that one of the reasons black men are at such a high risk for prostate cancer is because dark skin has a hard time absorbing vitamin D produced by the body after exposure to sunlight.

The best place to find vitamin D is outside, since sunlight is the only natural source. Because it is essential to health, a small amount of vitamin D is added to all dairy products and most breakfast cereals, but studies strongly suggest that much more is needed for optimal health.

Cancer, calcium, and vitamin D

Dairy products, the main dietary source of calcium, have consistently been linked to an increased risk of prostate cancer.

Multiple studies have found the risk is associated with doses of calcium in excess of 2,000 milligrams a day, but not in doses of 1,000 milligrams or less. One study reported in *Cancer Research* found consuming large amounts of calcium increased the risk of metastatic disease by 400 percent!

Vitamin D is necessary for the body to regulate calcium levels, so when taking a calcium supplement, it's wise to also take vitamin D.

Since vitamin D has anticancer properties, researchers aren't sure if calcium itself stimulates cancer growth, or if excess calcium lowers vitamin D levels and possibly interferes with the anticancer protective effects of vitamin D.

Quercetin: fighting prostate pain

Does your prostate give you pain? You might find relief with quercetin.

Quercetin is one of a group of powerful antioxidants called flavonoids that frequently get the credit for helping make a lot of fruits and vegetables super healthy. As a stand-alone nutrient, quercetin's roster of health claims is long. It fights infections, heart disease, cancer, allergies, and ulcers. It also offers men relief from the pelvic pain associated with chronic nonbacterial prostatitis.

A handful of small studies found that supplemental quercetin was powerful enough to ease unrelenting pain and urinary tract symptoms in men with severe chronic prostatitis. This is significant because nonbacterial prostatitis is a baffling disease and pharmaceutical drugs bring symptom relief to only about 50 percent of men who take them.

Doctors at the Cleveland Clinic found that taking quercetin supplements reduced symptoms in 84 percent of 100 men who volunteered to give it a try. After six months their scores dropped an average of six points — the barometer for success — on the Chronic Prostatitis Symptom Index (CPSI), a quality-of-life questionnaire that measures the severity of the disease. (You can find the CPSI on page 73). Another study at the Institute of Male Urology in Encino, California, found symptoms eased by 25 percent in 82 percent of men after taking quercetin twice a day for a month.

"Quercetin is well-tolerated and provides significant symptom improvement in most men with chronic pelvic pain," concluded doctors at the Cleveland Clinic.

Quercetin offers the prostate more than pain relief. Researchers are also looking into quercetin as a possible treatment for prostate cancer. Dozens of studies have found that the substance stops the proliferation of cancer cells and kills prostate tumors in the test tube.

Common sources of quercetin

Quercetin is a compound generously distributed through the plant kingdom. Apple peels are the best source, but it's found in many commonly consumed foods, including:

- berries
- cabbage
- seeds
- tea
- onions
- nuts

Green tea extract: getting EGCG the easy way

If you're not a green tea kind of a guy, you might be able to get the same prostate-protecting benefit you get from sipping tea all day by taking the extract as a supplement. And what you'll get is a con-centrated source of epigallocatechin gallate (EGCG), the all-important cell-protecting catechin that makes drinking tea so kind to the prostate.

When it comes to protecting the prostate, EGCG has a take-no-prisoners attitude. One study involved 60 Italian men with pre-malignant lesions in the prostate, a condition called high-grade prostatic intraepithelial neoplasia (HGPIN), that put them at high risk for cancer. They were put on either a capsule containing EGCG — the equivalent of drinking 16 cups of tea a day — or a placebo for one year. After one year, only 3 percent of the men taking the green tea extract were diagnosed with prostate cancer compared to 30 percent of the men who took the placebo. The trend continued well into the second year.

Among the same group of men, half also suffered from the urinary discomforts that go hand-in-hand with BPH, but they agreed not to undergo any treatment for the symptoms during the study. Sixty-five percent of them reported a "small but significant decrease" in urinary problems as a result of taking the extract, an effect the researchers contributed to the extract.

"Our findings suggest a new scenario in which the incidence of this disease could be greatly reduced by simply making [EGCG] available to the elderly or men at high risk," concluded the researchers in the journal *Cancer Research*. "The fact that no side or adverse effects have been reported confirms that [EGCG], at least in the dosage used here, is safe to humans."

In another study, researchers at Louisiana State University put 26 men ranging in age from 18 to 75 on an even higher dose of green tea extract daily for approximately one month before undergoing a radical prostatectomy. All biomarkers for cancer decreased and the men experienced modest reductions in PSA levels.

"These findings support a potential role of [green tea extract] in the treatment or prevention of prostate cancer," the researchers reported in *Cancer Prevention Research*.

In both studies, researchers believed the dosages were well tolerated because the type of supplement used was low in caffeine.

(Also see *Green Tea* on page 258.)

Curcumin: India's gift to prostate health

Curcumin is the active ingredient in turmeric, the brilliant deep yellow spice known as "Indian gold." Turmeric is so popular in India that it can be found in virtually every dish. What is hard to find in India, though, is prostate disease.

Indian men have the lowest incidence of prostate cancer in the world, and many researchers believe much of the credit belongs to the potent anti-inflammatory qualities of curcumin. Among them is Bharat B. Aggarwal, Ph.D., head of cancer research at University of Texas MD Anderson Cancer Center in Houston and the author of the book *Healing Spices*.

"Curcumin contains significant cancer-preventive and cancer-fighting characteristics," says Dr. Aggarwal, who is also the world's leading expert on curcumin. "It has been shown to fight prostate cancer on all levels." This includes some of the most aggressive and deadliest forms. And, it has been found to help prevent BPH.

Dr. Aggarwal has found that curcumin's anti-inflammatory capacity is so strong that it has the ability to interfere with the formation of what scientists call reactive oxygen species (ROS), the buildup of damaged cells that create the oxidative stress, or damage, that leads to serious and chronic health problems, such as cancer.

Thousands of studies have illustrated curcumin's cancer-fighting qualities and many of them have been on prostate cancer. Though curcumin has been found to inhibit a variety of cancers in human studies, human trials have yet to be conducted on prostate cancer, says Dr. Aggarwal. In *Healing Spices*, Dr. Aggarwal ticks off curcumin's cancer-fighting attributes. Studies have found that it can:

- inhibit the activation of genes that trigger cancer.

- kill cells that mutate into cancer.

- shrink tumors.

- prevent tumors from spreading to other organs.

- inhibit the transformation of normal cells into cancer cells.

- enhance the cancer-destroying effects of chemotherapy and radiation.

For example, the journal *Cancer Research* published a study in which scientists gave mice prostate cancer, then divided them into four different treatment groups. One group was treated with curcumin, a second received chemotherapy, a third got radiation, and the fourth received no treatment at all. Of the four, curcumin worked the best at controlling the disease.

When Korean researchers injected test animals with metastatic prostate cells, treatment with curcumin three times a week resulted in "significantly fewer" nodules that in animals given traditional treatment.

In a review in the journal *Cancer Letters*, Dr. Aggarwal reported on a man with a specific abnormality in the prostate gland called high-grade prostatic intraepithelial neoplasia (HGPIN), a condition that commonly leads to prostate cancer. The research team treated him three times a week for a year and a half with an herbal supplement containing curcumin. After six months, a biopsy showed no signs of HGPIN, even though the prostate was still enlarged. By 18 months, the prostate shrank back to normal size and was disease-free.

In a study at Rutgers University, researchers found a combined regimen of curcumin and isothiocyanate, the same substance that makes cabbage family vegetables prostate-protectors, reversed the growth of prostate tumors in mice.

Seeking curcumin: common curry misconception

Curcumin's only known source is the Indian spice turmeric. It is commonly believed that the best source of curcumin is curry powder, but this is a misconception. The curry powder found in the spice aisle of the supermarket is not a true spice at all, but a blend of spices that includes turmeric — and one shunned by Indian cooks. Its curcumin content is only as strong as the amount of turmeric in the curry mix, and this can vary from one product to the next. To get curcumin naturally, you should use the spice turmeric.

The curry powder you find in the supermarket is not an Indian spice; rather, it is an invention that originated in England. Curry in India is a method of cooking. Indian curries contain a variety of different spices, though the one essential ingredient is turmeric. Curry leaf is an Indian spice that bears no relationship to turmeric and contains no curcumin.

Even if you don't include turmeric in your regular cooking, you're probably getting more of it in your diet than you think. Turmeric is the spice that gives the bright yellow coloring to mustard. It also gives the yellow hue to canned chicken broth, butter, margarine, yellow cakes, bread-and-butter pickles, and popcorn.

African plum extract:
a capsule a day helps keep BPH away

African plum is to Central Africa what the apple is to America. Virtually everyone there loves it and eats it almost daily.

BPH is rare among Central African men and their fondness for the tangy taste of their favorite fruit is believed to be the reason why. Numerous studies during the last few decades have found that taking an extract made from the bark of the African plum tree appears to be just as effective as eating the real thing in helping to prevent BPH and the urinary tract symptoms that go with it.

When scientists in Minneapolis analyzed studies involving 1,562 men, they found that taking the extract "modestly, but significantly improved" urine flow and other urinary tract symptoms in men with BPH. Men who took the supplement were more than twice as likely to report a reduction in overall symptoms.

African plum contains powerful anti-inflammatory agents that work by inhibiting the production of prostaglandins, which produce the inflammation associated with an enlarged prostate. Scientists also believe constituents in African plum help reduce sensitivity in the bladder.

Although African plum is not as well-known in the United States in comparison to other natural remedies for BPH, it has been a popular treatment for more than 50 years in Germany, France, and many parts of Europe. It was first introduced to the Western world during the 1700s when travelers from Europe to Central Africa learned the fruit, known as *safou*, was a local cure for "old man's disease."

African plum is also known as *pygeum*, after its botanical name *Pygeum africanum*.

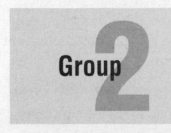

Group 2

These substances are supported by numerous animal studies, and perhaps limited human studies, with consistently promising results.

Lycopene: the prostate's little helper

When men look at an Italian menu, they see pizza and pasta. When cancer researchers look at an Italian menu, they see lycopene.

Lycopene is the substance that puts tomatoes at the top of the list of prostate-friendly foods. Lycopene, a member of a group of cancer-fighters called carotenoids, has been known as the "prostate nutrient" ever since researchers discovered that populations with a diet rich in tomatoes have a low incidence of prostate cancer.

Tomatoes and tomato products are the richest sources of lycopene, which is what led scientists to put one (lycopene) and one (tomatoes) together to see if they added up to a low rate of prostate cancer and BPH. They did. When they analyzed the diets of nearly 5,000 men participating in the long-term Prostate Cancer Prevention Trial, they found that men with the highest levels of lycopene in their blood had an 18 percent reduced risk of BPH.

Studies on supplemental lycopene and prostate cancer, however, have not been consistent. In fact, when researchers did a large-scale analysis of studies, they found the supplement appeared to offer some protection against all cancers except for prostate cancer. Subsequent research, however, has pinpointed a reason for this baffling finding. It appears lycopene is most effective when it gets help from other nutrients, as would typically be the case when it's consumed in many foods.

In one study, 500 Chinese men were divided into three groups. One group took lycopene supplements daily for several months. Another group drank green tea daily, and the third group took lycopene and drank green tea. Researchers found a reduced risk of prostate cancer in all three groups, but the men who took lycopene and drank green tea had the lowest risk of all.

Another study tested the power of supplemental lycopene and genistein, an isoflavone found in soy, on more than 70 men diagnosed with prostate cancer who had had three consecutive elevated PSA readings. The men were randomly selected to take lycopene alone or lycopene plus genistein twice a day for six months. Both groups experienced a drop in PSA levels, but the men taking lycopene plus genistein got the biggest benefit. A third study found taking lycopene supplements in conjunction with a low-fat, soy-based vegan diet slowed progression of disease in men with advanced prostate cancer.

Amazing but true: a natural cure

It's mighty rare for a man to check himself into hospice to die and later walk out alive — and well. But such was the case for a man in his late 60s who was dying of prostate cancer that had spread to his bones.

Doctors at the Comprehensive Cancer Center at Wake Forest University School of Medicine in Winston-Salem, North Carolina, first met the man in 1996 when he came to the hospital to be treated for recurring prostate cancer that had been diagnosed and treated five years earlier. The man had an extremely high PSA of 18.8, though tests confirmed the cancer had not spread.

Wake Forest doctors put him on hormone deprivation therapy to halt testosterone production, which they thought should have stopped or at least slowed the progress of the cancer, at least temporarily. Only it didn't — hormone deprivation therapy is often disappointing in aggressive prostate cancer. The doctors watched as the man's PSA rose to 43.6. They switched drugs, but to no avail. The man's PSA rose to 73. Other treatments failed as well and his PSA eventually rose to 365. Tests confirmed cancer had spread extensively and was in his bones. There was nothing more the doctors could do.

"The patient stopped all formal treatment regimens and transferred to hospice care," the doctors wrote in the August 2001 edition of the *Journal of Urology*. "In March 1999, he began taking lycopene and saw palmetto supplements." That's when the unexpected started to happen. "PSA decreased to 129.6 in April and to 8.1 in May. PSA remained from 3 to 8 for 18 months." A repeat bone scan showed there was less cancer in his bone. "At last follow-up," they reported two years later, "he was asymptomatic."

Though the man had taken both lycopene and saw palmetto, the doctors gave all the credit to lycopene, because multiple studies showed that saw palmetto failed to lower PSA in men. They had no other comment.

Finding lycopene in food

Tomatoes and tomato products by far are the richest source of lycopene. You'll find measurably more lycopene in a can of tomato sauce than a fresh tomato because lycopene activity increases with cooking. Other good sources of lycopene include:

- apricots
- grapefruit
- papayas
- watermelon
- asparagus
- guavas
- sweet red peppers

Resveratrol: wine in a capsule

Resveratrol is the rare polyphenol antioxidant and anti-inflammatory substance that gets most of the credit for turning the ritual of having a daily glass or two of wine with dinner into a laudable health habit.

Though resveratrol is best-known as a compound that's good for the heart, researchers are hot on the trail associating it with a laundry list of health conditions, including a dozen forms of cancer. One of them is prostate cancer. Though studies to date have been limited to the lab and animals, researchers are getting promising results.

A plethora of lab tests have found that resveratrol halts human prostate cancer cell lines at initiation, promotion, and progression stages of even the most aggressive forms of the disease. A limited number of studies are finding the same results in test mice with cancer that closely mimics human prostate cancer. In one study, reported in the journal *Carcinogenesis*, researchers found resveratrol reduced progression of high-grade prostate cancer in test mice by 62 percent, making the researchers speculate that there is "a potential for resveratrol in the diet to protect against spontaneously developing prostate cancer."

Searching for dietary resveratrol

Most resveratrol is found in the skin of grapes, which is why wine, and most specifically red wine, is the richest dietary source of resveratrol. The skin is included in making red wine but is removed in making white wine. Since drinking wine is not a choice for everyone, you may want to get your resveratrol another way. The supplement Resvinatrol contains, among other natural sources of resveratrol, muscadine grape blend and muscadine grape seed extract. Drink one ounce of the liquid form to get 100 milligrams of resvera-trol, more than would be available in a large bottle of grape juice or red wine. Check out the products online at *www.resvinatrol complete.com.*

Supplements containing dry powdered extracts of resveratrol may have questionable benefits. Grape juice, red wine, or the liquid Resvinatrol product are more natural, like the foods containing reveratrol that are shown to be beneficial in many studies.

Food sources of resveratrol include:

- blueberries
- mulberries
- grapes and grape juice
- peanuts

Fish oil: striving for balance

If you don't care for fish and don't eat it at least twice a week, then you might want to consider taking a daily fish oil supplement. Dozens of studies suggest that it may offer your prostate the same protection as eating a healthy fish dinner.

It's not fish itself, but the omega-3 fatty acids found in fatty types of fish that are so good for your prostate — and your heart, too. Omega-3 fatty acids are polyunsaturated fats that the body needs but cannot manufacture. A chief source is fatty fish. Studies suggest about two servings of fish a week are all it takes to offer protection against prostate cancer.

Several population studies, including one that followed more than 6,000 men for 30 years, suggest that either eating fish or taking fish oil supplements reduces the risk of prostate cancer.

Taking fish oil supplements has been found to be beneficial to men undergoing chemotherapy for advanced prostate cancer. Studies found that men who took fish oil supplements experienced few side effects and it helped enhance the effectiveness of the drugs, thus improving the chances of a better outcome.

"In combination with standard treatment, supplementing the diet with fatty acids may be a nontoxic means to improve cancer treatment outcomes and may slow or prevent recurrence of cancer," reported researchers at Louisiana State University, who reviewed all the literature in relation to cancer treatment and omega-3 fatty acids. "Used alone, a supplement may be a useful alternative therapy for patients who are not candidates for standard toxic cancer therapies."

A balancing act

Scientists proved the importance of getting enough omega-3s in the diet when they looked at a nutritional imbalance in the American diet that may be contributing to the high rate of prostate cancer in the United States. The typical Western diet contains a disproportionate amount of omega-3 fatty acids to omega-6 fatty acids, say scientists at the Center for Genetics, Nutrition and Health in Washington. Omega-6 fatty acids are found in oils, such as safflower, sunflower, and palm.

When the researchers measured the ratio of omega-6 to omega-3 in a group of American men, they found the average to be 10:1. In some men it was as high as 30:1! For optimal health, the ratio is 4:1.

Why is this so important? Because studies indicate that omega-3s protect against prostate disease while omega-6s contribute to it. In one study, blood levels of omega-3s were significantly lower in men with BPH and prostate cancer and levels of omega-6s were significantly higher.

Making fish oil taste better

Some men complain that they don't like taking fish oil supplements because they leave a fishy aftertaste. If you've had this experience, try these strategies recommended by the Mayo Clinic.

Take it at mealtime. Taking fish oil with food can help buffer the odor.

Try an odorless supplement. Coated capsules actually pass through the stomach and dissolve in the intestines.

Switch brands. Some manufacturers make a pure omega-3 fatty acid product that doesn't taste fishy, although it is likely to cost more than standard products.

Swallow the capsule frozen. This slows the breakdown of fish oil in the stomach, which reduces fishy burps. It will not affect digestion or absorption of the supplement.

Major sources of fish oil

Not all fish are good sources of omega-3s. The oil is found in fatty fish that generally roam cold water. The main sources of omega-3s are:

▪ albacore white tuna	▪ anchovies
▪ cod	▪ halibut
▪ herring	▪ lake trout
▪ salmon	▪ striped bass

Note that wild-caught Alaskan salmon, available in many brands of canned salmon, has, by far, the least amount of toxins of all fish products. (Also see *Fish*, page 253.)

Pectin: modified to fight cancer

Pectin is a type of soluble fiber present in many plants, but it is concentrated in the peel and pulp of apples, pears, and citrus fruit. Modified citrus pectin (MCP) is an altered form that is more absorbable than the natural pectin in fruit. It's important to prostate health because it possesses strong anti-cancer properties.

MCP has attracted the attention of researchers because laboratory studies have found that it stops the proliferation of cancer cells and can kill even the most aggressive prostate tumors. As a result, a study is currently underway in California in which modified forms of pectin are being used to treat men with advanced cancer that does not respond well to treatment. Phase two of the study involved 13 men who had a recurrence of prostate cancer after being treated through radical prostatectomy, radiation therapy, or cryosurgery. After one year of treatment, 70 percent of the men experienced a slowdown in their PSA doubling time, a sign that the progression of disease had slowed.

Researchers believe pectin contains yet-to-be-identified compounds that stop and kill cancer more effectively than currently available medications. Researchers at the University of Georgia believe there is "a basis for the development of pectin-based pharmaceuticals, nutraceuticals, or recommended diet changes aimed at combating prostate cancer occurrence and progression."

Dietary choices for pectin

As a type of fiber, pectin is plentiful in the plant food kingdom. It's the gel that makes fruit jellies so gooey. Some of the top sources of pectin are:

- apples
- beans
- carrots
- celery
- cucumbers
- grapefruit
- oranges
- peas
- tomatoes

Grape seed extract: a wine alternative

Grape seed extract (GSE), a byproduct of fermented wine, is a super-saturated source of a complex mixture of antioxidants. Among its claim to fame: It is 20 times more potent than vitamin C and 50 times more powerful than vitamin E — facts that contribute to its association with reducing the risk of 43 different health problems.

The substance that makes grape seed extract really stand out as something special to the prostate is gallic acid, a polyphenol believed to be exceptionally effective at protecting prostate cells from the oxidative damage that leads to cancer.

Several studies in mice during the last decade found that GSE can fight all types of prostate cancer — even the most lethal — on multiple levels. It can kill cancer cells, arrest tumor growth, and stop tumors from spreading to other organs.

In one study, researchers from the University of Colorado Health Sciences Center inoculated test mice with prostate cancer cells, which caused many to develop high-grade prostatic intraepithelial neoplasia (HGPIN), a condition that usually leads to cancer. Feeding the mice grape seed extract resulted in "a strong reduction" in the incidence of cancer, even among the mice with the most advanced HGPIN.

Researchers in Japan found the same effect when they used grape seed extract to fight human metastatic prostate cells that are resistant to conventional treatment.

Exactly how grape seed extract defends the prostate had eluded experts until researchers at the University of Kentucky figured it out. It appears substances in the extract work together to sniff out and "wake up" a specific protein called JNK that prompts damaged prostate cells to self-destruct.

Seeking gallic acid naturally

Wine, both red and white, is the most potent source of gallic acid. It is found in minute amounts in other plant foods. Among the other sources are:

- apple seeds
- bananas
- grape seeds
- lemons
- pineapples
- strawberries

Beta-sitosterol: helps with urinary control

Beta-sitosterol, a plant fat found in fruits, vegetables, nuts, and seeds, is used in the United States in medications that fight certain health problems, including heart disease and high cholesterol. BPH, however, is not among them — at least not yet. But beta-sitosterol is being used in Germany and other parts of Europe as a stand-alone prostate drug, reportedly with great success, as a result of a handful of successful studies showing it reduced lower urinary tract difficulties and improved the quality of life in men with BPH.

In one study, reported in the British medical journal *Lancet*, researchers gave 200 men with BPH either a beta-sitosterol supplement or a placebo. After six months, the men taking the supplement showed a noticeable decline in all symptoms, which were measured using the International Prostate Symptom Score (IPSS), which rates the severity of BPH and its impact on quality of life. (You can find the IPSS on page 43). The beneficial effect lasted for an additional 18 months after the men stopped taking the supplement. Those taking a placebo experienced no improvement in symptoms.

"Significant improvement in symptoms and urinary flow parameters show the effectiveness of beta-sitosterol in the treatment of benign prostatic hyperplasia," the researchers concluded.

In another study, reported in the *British Journal of Urology*, 117 men with BPH reported similar results, although they did not find the positive effects lasted after supplementation stopped. Their improvement was noticeable enough to the men who got the placebo pill that they, too, volunteered to take the supplement. "They improved to the extent of the treated group on all outcomes," the researchers reported.

Food sources of beta-sitosterol

Beta-sitosterol is widely available in all plant foods. It is found in vegetable oils and margarine. However, it should not be confused with sitosterol, the substance found in the nondairy spread Benecol. Main food sources of beta-sitosterol include:

- almonds
- avocados
- canola oil
- corn oil
- fava beans
- grape leaves
- margarine
- pistachios
- soy beans
- vegetable oil

Black cumin: the seed of good health

Unless you've been to India or are seriously into Indian cooking, chances are you never heard of black cumin seeds. These glistening tiny flecks, black as coal, are so popular in India they are used in everything from chutneys and curries to yogurt dishes and breads. As popular as they are as a spice, black cumin seeds are revered even more for their healing power.

Scientists around the world are scrutinizing black cumin as a possible treatment for more than a dozen types of cancer, including prostate cancer. They are finding that it is so powerful it has the ability to attack prostate cancer on all levels. The focus of interest is the oil found in the seeds, containing a tongue-twister of an antioxidant called thymoquinone — or, as researchers call it for short, TQ. The compound is so unique it is yet to be detected in any other plant. Researchers believe that TQ may be part of the reason why men in India have the lowest rate of prostate cancer in the world.

Research is still new and scientists aren't yet sure how it works, but they know that it can stimulate natural killer cells in the immune system to detect and destroy cancer cells. Researchers at Henry Ford Hospital in Michigan found that TQ blocked cellular receptors for the hormones that power the growth of prostate tumors. "We conclude that thymoquinone, a naturally occurring herbal product, may prove to be effective in treating … prostate cancer," they reported in the journal *Cancer Research*. "Furthermore," they continued, "because of its selective effect on cancer cells, we believe that thymoquinone can also be used safely to help prevent the development of prostate cancer."

Where to find black cumin

TQ is as obscure in health food stores as black cumin seeds are in the spice section of the average supermarket. However, if you have access to an Indian market you should be able to find black cumin as a spice or black cumin oil as a medicinal tincture.

Black cumin seeds are inexpensive and very healthy. They are a bastion of important nutrients, including eight out of nine essential amino acids, essential fatty acids, beta carotene, calcium, iron, and potassium. In all, more than 100 chemicals important to health have been identified in black cumin seeds, and researchers believe many more are yet to be discovered.

You'll find the taste reminiscent of that hard-to-detect flavor that makes Indian chutneys and the flatbread called *naan* so distinct.

Black cumin has no relationship to the popular spices cumin or curcumin, either botanically or medicinally.

Lupeol: medicinal mango

In India the tropical fruit mango is revered as "the king of all fruit," so it's no surprise that Indians were the first to discover that its most exotic component, lupeol, is a potent anti-cancer agent.

Animal research shows that lupeol, a phytosterol, can stop progression of a number of hard-to-cure cancers, including the most lethal form of prostate cancer. When test mice were fed lupeol, researchers discovered it stopped the development and proliferation of human prostate cells without harming healthy cells. The more lupeol the mice ate, the greater the nutrient's anti-cancer effect.

In one recent experiment, scientists injected male mice with enough testosterone to make the prostate grow. For the next two weeks, half the mice received supplemental lupeol in their mouse chow; the other half got no lupeol. Meanwhile, they watched to see what happened. They saw prostates grow in the lupeol-deprived mice, but not in the mice fed lupeol.

Said researchers at the University of Wisconsin, "We suggest that lupeol could be developed as a potential agent for the treatment of human prostate cancer."

Lupeol: it's everywhere

There is no shortage of lupeol in food and you should be getting your fair share if you are eating plenty of fruits and vegetables. Lupeol is found in a wide variety of plant foods, including cereals and plant-based oils. Lupeol is found in a variety of vegetables and fruits, including:

- cabbage
- cucumbers
- figs
- mangoes
- olives
- strawberries
- tomatoes

Black cohosh:
relief for symptoms of advanced disease

News flash: Black cohosh is not the exclusive domain of women's health anymore.

This inedible herb, well-known for decades as the herb to quell hot flashes in women going through menopause, is now targeting men's health — and it's aimed right for the prostate gland.

Hot flashes are common in men who are going through hormone deprivation therapy, also known as androgen ablation therapy, as a treatment for advanced prostate cancer, only they are much worse than in the typical woman going through menopause.

Black cohosh's medicinal power comes from its ability to emit estrogen-like signals — the key to its knack in knocking back menopausal hot flashes. So if it works for women, wondered researchers, could it also help men experiencing hot flashes as a result of going through hormone deprivation therapy for prostate cancer? The conclusion they came to was yes. Several studies have found that it can be just as effective in men as it is in women.

One study at the Mayo Clinic found that five weeks of treatment with black cohosh cut the frequency of hot flashes from six times a day to two and significantly reduced the severity of the heat. Doctors in Germany are experimenting with black cohosh in helping to prevent bone loss and osteoporosis, which are other side effects of the hormone therapy.

Though research is fairly new and less than 10 studies have been conducted, researchers are also investigating this herb as a prostate cancer preventive.

In one study, reported in the journal *Pharmacology*, researchers injected one million cancer cells into the prostates of 36 test mice. Half the animals were put on a diet containing black cohosh. The chow fed to the other mice did not contain the herb. Two months after the inoculation, 12 of 18 mice on the herb-free diet developed solid masses in the prostate. Only five of the 18 mice given black cohosh developed cancer "and the size of the tumors [was] significantly smaller." This led the researchers to conclude that black cohosh "may prove to be effective in the prevention and treatment of prostate cancer."

A similar study, reported in *Anti-Cancer Research*, called black cohosh "a novel therapeutic approach for the treatment of prostate cancer."

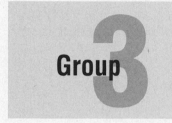

Group 3

These supplements are the subject of new research with limited but positive scientific results in animal and test tube studies, or are controversial due to conflicting evidence.

Vitamin E: protective oil

The role of vitamin E in prostate health is confusing. For years, many men depended on vitamin E supplements as insurance against prostate disease based on evidence that it reduced the risk of prostate cancer in smokers.

The study, involving 29,000 smokers, found taking vitamin E supplements reduced the incidence of prostate cancer by 32 percent and decreased the risk of dying from prostate cancer by 41 percent. Other studies found the effect to be as high as 50 percent. One study found that even a small dose of vitamin E was better than taking no vitamin E.

A more recent follow-up study involving 47,780 professionals in the United States, however, has muddied the thinking about the true role of vitamin E in prostate disease. The study confirmed that vitamin E was protective against prostate cancer in men who smoked or recently quit smoking, but not in nonsmokers.

Even more confusing was another study finding "excessive" intake of vitamin E may be causing more harm than good. The researchers, reporting in the *Annals of Internal Medicine*, found that taking 400 IU daily, the amount found in many over-the-counter supplements, appeared to increase the risk of death from prostate cancer. Another study, reported in the *New England Journal of Medicine*, also found that taking the supplement decreased the effectiveness of cholesterol-lowering drugs.

The key to understanding these conflicting results may lie in the form of vitamin E that was used in most of these studies — alpha-tocopherol. When physicians studied the use of gamma-tocopherol instead of alpha-tocopherol, they found a very powerful effect in preventing prostate cancer.

Getting the most vitamin E

So what to do? There is plenty of evidence showing that foods high in natural vitamin E are protective against prostate cancer, perhaps because these foods contain more than one tocopherol, including gamma.

Vitamin E is a hard-working antioxidant, though it isn't all that easy to get from food, mostly because it is primarily found in nuts and vegetable oils. The largest dietary source is wheat germ. In addition, you can look for vitamin E in these foods:

almonds	mangoes	turnips
peanuts	walnuts	vegetable oils

Zinc: an aphrodisiac for prostate health

Eat oysters, love longer.

This timeless expression was born out of the oyster's well-known reputation as an aphrodisiac. History tells us that the dashing lover

Casanova started his evening meal by eating dozens of oysters! It's not such a far-fetched idea if prostate health is your goal.

If researchers could have dissected Casanova's prostate, they might have learned something about prostate disease. Oysters are, by far, the largest dietary source of zinc, a trace mineral that's attracted to the prostate. Zinc is important to prostate health. Studies show that cancerous prostates contain much less zinc than healthy prostates, evidence that suggests increased zinc is associated with a lower incidence of prostate disease.

Results of the Prostate Cancer Prevention Trial found that men with the highest dietary and supplemental zinc levels had a 32 percent reduced risk of developing BPH compared to men with the lowest zinc counts.

Zinc's role in preventing prostate cancer, however, is controversial — at least supplemental zinc. Although several studies have found that high levels of zinc can stop human cancer cell growth in the test tube, a recent population study found that men who were taking high levels of zinc supplements for at least 10 years were at increased risk for prostate cancer. However, researchers noted that these men were taking toxic levels of the mineral.

Nevertheless, researchers at Oregon State University, where much of the prostate and zinc studies are being conducted, are high on zinc's potential as a prostate protector. In a recent review, they noted that "studies suggest that zinc may play an important role in regulating the cell growth that leads to both prostate cancer and BPH."

Think zinc foods

Zinc, however, is an essential mineral. It helps protect DNA from oxidative damage and assists in DNA repair. Statistics show that 70 percent of American men do not get enough zinc to maintain basic prostate health. You can find zinc in these foods without the danger of overdosing with supplements:

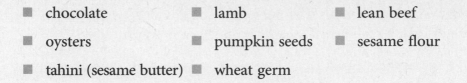

- chocolate
- lamb
- lean beef
- oysters
- pumpkin seeds
- sesame flour
- tahini (sesame butter)
- wheat germ

Beta carotene: not the final word

At one time, supplemental beta carotene was practically synonymous with cancer prevention, but that's not the case any longer. Not only is its ability to help prevent cancer in question, some studies have actually found beta carotene supplementation is associated with an increased cancer risk.

Fueling the controversy was a 2009 study involving more than 77,000 Americans that found long-term use of beta carotene supplements was associated with an increased risk of cancer among smokers. Another study found that long-term beta carotene supplementation decreased the effectiveness of cancer treatments, but also in smokers.

So what if you're not a smoker? The evidence is muddled here, too. Though there are some 20 studies showing that men with high blood levels of beta carotene had a lower risk for prostate cancer, there are even more studies showing beta carotene has no impact at all on the incidence of prostate cancer. Some studies suggest it could increase the risk of aggressive cancer.

It's a controversy that has a lot of nutrition "experts" who had recommended taking beta carotene scratching their heads and wondering, so what gives? One explanation says beta carotene is so effective that years of supplementation causes a boomerang effect and it actually turns on itself. Another is that it simply doesn't mix well with nicotine.

Beta carotene is a highly active antioxidant belonging to a family of cancer-fighting nutrients known as carotenoids. It is of keen interest among nutritionists and researchers because it is one of the substances that provides the deep rich color to green and orange fruits and vegetables — and one of the nutritional reasons we are encouraged to eat them. However, there appears to be a difference between eating fruits and vegetables rich in beta carotene and taking beta carotene supplements. Supplements appear to miss something important associated with getting nutrients naturally from food.

A large study published in the *International Journal of Cancer* in 2010 attempted to get to the bottom of the controversy. "This study adds to the evidence that nutritional prevention of cancer through beta carotene supplementation should not be recommended," the study's author concluded. Most likely, however, this will not be the final word.

Beta carotene by the bunch

There is no shortage of carotene in our food supply, not just beta carotene, but many related substances. These carotenes are in many of the fruits and vegetables that have been found to promote prostate health. For example, spinach, a top pro-prostate food, is one of the richest sources of beta carotene. Other sources include:

- apricots
- broccoli
- butternut squash
- cantaloupe
- carrots
- collard greens
- kale
- mango
- papaya
- pumpkin
- sweet potatoes

Vitamin C: cast in controversy

Ever since Linus Pauling claimed that high doses of vitamin C could prevent cancer nearly 50 years ago, the role this popular and common nutrient plays in cancer control has been cast in controversy.

When Pauling was diagnosed with prostate cancer in 1993 he claimed his high intake of vitamin C supplements had kept his disease at bay for 20 years. He died from the cancer a year later at the age of 93.

During the last several decades, thousands of studies have been conducted on vitamin C and cancer. For every study that says vitamin C helps prevent cancer there is another one that says taking vitamin C supplements is a waste of time.

Though there are several studies that show vitamin C can stop prostate tumors from proliferating in Petri dishes and test animals, studies involving thousands of men who take vitamin C supplements indicate it has no affect on a man's risk of getting cancer or BPH. On the other hand, one large population study found that eating foods rich in vitamin C, but not taking vitamin C supplements, is protective against prostate cancer.

Seeking vitamin C

The bottom line? Prostate cancer specialists take a conservative point of view on vitamin C. It's an essential and important vitamin that is best to get through food. This is easy enough, as scores of fruits and vegetables, are rich in vitamin C, especially citrus fruits. These are among the best sources:

- bell peppers
- broccoli
- Brussels sprouts
- citrus fruit
- kale
- kiwi
- sweet potatoes
- tomatoes

Conjugated linoleic acid: a good fat for the prostate

Conjugated linoleic acid, better known as CLA, is not your ordinary good-for-you fat. For one, its healing action comes from a unique combination of compounds called isomers that are popular with the beauty industry as a component in anti-wrinkle creams and with the diet industry as a slimming aid. For another, CLA is found in animal fat — the kind of fat suspected of contributing to prostate disease.

While CLA's role as a wrinkle eraser and dietary aid is controversial, its potential as a prostate protector is not. "CLA is an effective inhibitor of many human cancers, including prostate cancer," researchers reported in the journal *Carcinogenesis*. Studies have found that the isomers in CLA are powerful antioxidants that may have the ability to prevent prostate tumors from forming and reduce the size of existing tumors. When a research team from several European countries reviewed the studies on CLA and prostate disease, it concluded that "CLA could be a novel dietary supplement for individuals with increased risk of prostate cancer or patients undergoing prostate cancer treatment."

Noted another group of researchers from Argentina, "CLAs are the only natural fatty acids accepted by the National Academy of Sciences of the USA as exhibiting consistent anti-tumor properties at levels as low as 0.25 to 1 percent of total fats."

This can be translated to mean it doesn't take a lot of CLA to get a prostate-protecting effect.

Food sources of CLA

Researchers fall short of recommending supplements as your sole source of CLA, as there is the belief that the natural CLA in animal fat is far superior to synthetic CLA. This, however, is not a prescription for you to go hog-wild over eating fatty food.

For starters, CLA is quite choosy about where it resides. Its best food sources are the fat in raw dairy products and grass-fed animals — among them cows, goats, sheep, llamas, deer, and kangaroo. Kangaroo, by far, is the best food source of CLA, containing as much as 500 percent more CLA than what is found in grain-fed cattle. Raw dairy products and meat from grass-fed animals are difficult, if not impossible, to come by.

Researchers say your best bet for getting CLA naturally is by eating lean meat and low-fat dairy products, including milk, eggs, and small amounts of cheese. You should still trim the visible fat from steaks and chops. CLA is found in the invisible fat that extends through the muscle fibers of meat.

Selenium: protection — for some?

This trace mineral, which we get from food grown in selenium-rich soil, has been having an on-again, off-again rendezvous with cancer researchers ever since they first started to notice a correlation between selenium deficiency in the diet and the risk of certain cancers, including prostate cancer. They observed that in parts of the world where selenium content in soil is low, rates of prostate cancer are high, and in areas where soil is rich in selenium, cancer rates are low.

Selenium's prostate protection is believed to come from special antioxidants called selenoproteins that attack cancer cells by cutting off their blood supply, essentially causing them to suffocate and die.

During the 1990s, several studies kindled the hope that taking selenium supplements would help reduce the risk of prostate cancer. One study of 1,300 American men found that taking selenium daily reduced cancer rates by 41 percent after 10 years. Another study found that men with high blood levels of selenium had a 39 percent lower risk of the disease. When Canadian researchers analyzed the results of 16 studies linking prostate cancer and selenium they concluded that men who took selenium supplements reduced their risk by an average of 28 percent. Yet another study found selenium was only protective when levels of vitamin E were also high.

These tantalizing findings led to a large study, called the Selenium and Vitamin E Cancer Prevention Trial (SELECT). It involved 35,000 men age 50 and older who took either 200 micrograms of selenium, 400 International Units (IU) of vitamin E, a combination of both, or a placebo. The results were disappointing. After four to seven years, men taking supplements were no less likely to get prostate cancer than the men taking the placebo.

Researchers aren't sure why SELECT produced such disappointing results after so many promising studies, but recent research at the Harvard School of Public Health suggests the reason some men benefit from selenium more than others is genetic. Despite conflicting evidence, some prostate specialists think selenium is beneficial, especially for men at high risk.

Finding selenium-rich foods

Selenium, which the body needs in small amounts — the daily value (DV) is 70 micrograms — comes from animals that graze on and plants that are grown in soil where the selenium is found naturally. The most selenium-rich soil in the United States is found in northern Nebraska and the high plains of the Dakotas. Selenium deficiency in the United States is not a problem because food distribution throughout the country literally spreads the mineral around. By contrast, selenium deficiency is a problem in parts of the world dependent on local crops for food. This occurs mostly in impoverished nations.

Brazil nuts by far contain more selenium than any other food. Just 1 ounce offers 780 percent of the DV. No other foods offer the DV in a single dose. In addition to Brazil nuts, selenium is generally found in these foods:

- beef
- cod
- cottage cheese
- eggs
- pasta
- turkey
- white tuna

Aged garlic extract: concentrated prostate protection?

Garlic is a culinary jewel of the Mediterranean diet and aged garlic extract is a concentrated source of prostate-protecting organosulfurs, the substance that makes the "stinking rose" so healthy. And it has a beneficent social bonus: It offers the healthy benefits of garlic without the residual reminder of what you ate at your last meal.

Aged garlic extract, or AGE for short, is extracted from fresh garlic bulbs that have been left to sit at room temperature for 20 months. This is said to help garlic's well-known anti-cancer properties multiply. During this aging time, harsh unstable compounds may gradually convert into stable, health-promoting substances.

Several studies have found that a specific substance in organosulfurs called diallyl disulfide (DADS) suppresses cancer growth and kills damaged prostate cells before they become cancerous. One laboratory study in China found DADS could inhibit the growth of damaged human prostate cells by 80 percent. Studies also show it can be helpful in diminishing the symptoms of BPH.

AGE also contains flavonoids, antioxidants with well-known cancer-fighting power, and the prostate-protecting mineral selenium. In fact, one study found that the organosulfurs and selenium in aged garlic work together to guard against prostate cancer better than either substance alone.

(Also see *Garlic* on page 244.)

Ellagic acid: support for chemotherapy

When you eat a bowl of berries, munch on a handful of walnuts, or quaff a glass of pomegranate juice, your prostate gets an injection of ellagic acid, a mighty potent antioxidant belonging to a special group of cancer-fighting compounds called polyphenols.

Ellagic acid appears to have special talent when it comes to treating prostate cancer. It can do what chemotherapy drugs can't do — discriminate between healthy and harmful cells. This is significant because chemotherapy drugs can kill mutant cells, but they destroy healthy cells as well. Ellagic acid, however, has the ability to destroy cancer cells without harming healthy cells. Initially, this ability was only observed in test-tube and animal studies, but recent research indicates it might work the same way in men with prostate cancer.

In one experiment, researchers in Italy put a group of men with prostate cancer on two different treatment regimens. One group was put on two chemotherapy drugs, and the other group was given the same drugs along with a large dose of ellagic acid. The men who were taking the ellagic acid experienced less damage to healthy cells as a result of the chemotherapy compared to the men who did not take the supplement. They also had stronger white cell counts than the men who did not get the supplement. Taking the supplement, noted the researchers, offered the men "a better biological outcome and better quality of life."

"Our study suggests that the use of ellagic acid as support therapy reduces chemotherapy-induced toxicity," reported the researchers in the journal *European Urology*.

Getting ellagic acid from food

More than 45 different fruits, nuts, and vegetables contain ellagic acid. Berries are the richest sources with red raspberries by far containing the most. Red raspberries contain more than twice the ellagic acid of any other food. Other top sources of ellagic acid are:

- cranberries
- pecans
- pomegranates
- strawberries
- walnuts

Red clover:
an experimental herb of interest

Alternative healers have been using red clover for more than 100 years as a medicinal herb to treat a host of ailments, including cancer — a fact that has not escaped the attention of the National Cancer Institute (NCI). When NCI scientist Jonathan Hartwell, Ph.D., researched the use of this herb as a cancer treatment several years ago, he discovered that healers in 33 different cultures around the world were using it. So Dr. Hartwell took red clover into his own lab and came out a believer.

Red clover, he found, is a rich source of potent isoflavones, most notably genistein and daidzein, two substances that get the credit for making soy foods so beneficial to the prostate. Scores of animal and laboratory tests from around the world have come to the same conclusion: red clover helps fight BPH and prostate cancer. Success in humans, however, is mostly anecdotal.

One small study in Australia tested the herb in a small group of men who were about to undergo a radical prostatectomy for early- or inter-mediate-grade prostate cancer. The men agreed to take red clover as a supplement for 20 days prior to surgery. When pathologists examined the tissue in the extracted prostates after the surgery, they found many of the cancer cells that had been active at biopsy were dead.

Animal studies show that red clover can stop the rise of out-of-control hormones that are suspected of causing the prostate to grow and cancer cells to proliferate. "This study suggests that dietary supple-mentation with red clover isoflavones may provide a nontoxic dietary treatment for prostatic hyperplasia with a concomitant reduction in the potential for development of prostate cancer," conclude the researchers from The University of Sydney in Australia.

Genistein: more than a hill of beans

Genistein, the active ingredient in soy foods, is proving to be bigger than a hill of beans when it comes to fighting prostate cancer.

Genistein is the most biologically active member of a well-known family of cancer-fighting antioxidants called isoflavones. Initially, numerous laboratory studies found genistein stopped growth of and caused death to human prostate cancer cell lines, as well as several other forms of cancer. Now, researchers are investigating genistein for its ability to help enhance radiation therapy used to treat metastatic prostate cancer.

In one experiment, researchers gave genistein to animals two days prior to giving them radiation treatment for prostate cancer that had spread to the lymph nodes. The treatment proved to be 87 percent effective. The same therapy in animals not pretreated with genistein was only 73 percent effective. Even treatment with genistein alone had a 30 percent success rate.

"Long-term therapy with genistein after prostate tumor irradiation significantly increased survival," noted the researchers in *Molecular Cancer Therapeutics*.

Caution: Soy products are loaded with genistein. Consuming large amounts of soy was associated with a high risk of developing dementia in elderly Hawaiians of Japanese ancestry.

On the search for genistein

Soy foods are the richest and most popular source of dietary genistein, but the nutrient is also present in other vegetables and vegetarian protein choices including:

■ beans   ■ lentils   ■ peas

(Also see *Soy* on page 269.)

Rye grass pollen extract: sleep better at night

The gut reaction on hearing the words grass pollen is to steer clear of it. Rye grass pollen may be the exception, if you have troublesome symptoms caused by BPH or prostatitis.

Rye grass pollen has been used as a natural prostate disease remedy ever since a Swedish researcher named Erick Ask-Upmark found that men who took rye grass pollen found relief from the symptoms of hard-to-treat chronic nonbacterial prostatitis nearly 40 years ago.

Since then, research studies have been few and far between. Two small studies involving 144 men found that taking rye grass pollen in a product known as Cernilton modestly improved symptoms, most notably by reducing the number of times the men had to get up in the middle of the night to urinate.

A study published in the *British Journal of Urology* found that 78 percent of men taking one supplement three times a day for six months found relief from the symptoms of chronic prostatitis, including pain. Of them, 36 percent reported being cured.

The research suggests that rye grass pollen works by relaxing the muscles of the urethra and improving the ability of the bladder to contract.

The U.S. Food and Drug Administration remains skeptical about rye grass pollen as an effective home remedy for the urinary symptoms and pain associated with these two conditions. You should not try this remedy if you are allergic to any types of grasses.

Fisetin: a possible healer on the horizon?

Researchers call it "novel," and you'd be hard pressed to even find it in a health food store, but fisetin is on the list of nutrients most likely to have a major impact on prostate health.

Why? Because fisetin may be one of the most powerful members of the cancer-fighting family of plant compounds called flavonoids. At least a dozen studies have found it is an antioxidant with potent anti-cancer activity. Researchers who found that fisetin killed and inhibited progression of human prostate cancer cells in test-tube experiments called the findings "significant."

One study teamed fisetin with bicalutamide (Casodex), a drug used to treat advanced prostate cancer, and found it enhanced the medicine's ability to stop the spread of prostate cancer. "Fisetin," researchers reported in *Molecular Cell Biochemistry*, "can serve as a potential candidate for treating cancer metastasis."

Seeking fisetin in food

Most of the scientific research on fisetin has been done on its ability to enhance memory and brain function. As a result, it is most commonly packaged in anti-aging formulations. It is not yet available as a stand-alone nutrient. Fisetin, however, is found in minute amounts in some fruits and vegetables. The top food sources of fisetin include:

- apples
- cucumbers
- onions
- persimmons
- strawberries

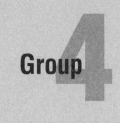

Group These supplements may be effective against certain prostate disorders, but because they inhibit testosterone production, they can cause significant adverse side effects, including reduced energy and decreased sexual desire.

Bee pollen extract: a honey of a symptom fighter

The stuff that bees gather to make honey and use to reproduce is loaded with vitamins, minerals, antioxidants, and other important nutrients essential to human health — a formula that appears to influence prostate health.

Studies show that bee pollen extract — particularly a certain kind called Cernitin, a special preparation made from eight different kinds of pollen — is so effective it is now being used experimentally with success in Europe and Japan to treat various diseases of the prostate, including BPH and nonbacterial prostatitis. Here are some of the findings.

- After taking bee pollen for six months, 79 percent of men with BPH reported a significant reduction in the need to urinate during the night, and 36 percent reported all symptoms of BPH had disappeared, according to a British study.

- Three months of bee pollen supplementation produced "favorable results" in older men with BPH, according to a Japanese study, and symptoms did not return after supplementation ended.

- In another experiment, also in Japan, researchers reported an overall success rate of 80 percent in men taking bee pollen extract. Among these men, 92 percent experienced a reduction in spontaneous urine leakage, 86 percent experienced improvement in urine stream and flow, 85 percent reported a reduced need to urinate during the night, and 56 percent found they no longer felt the need to strain during urination.

■ Doctors in Germany found that six months of treatment with Cernitin produced favorable results in men with chronic prostatitis. Among them, 36 percent were cured of symptoms and signs of the disease.

Researchers believe bee pollen works like many other treatments, by controlling the release of dihydrotestosterone, the active form of testosterone that doctors believe incites prostate disease. Low activity of testosterone is associated with reduced sexuality. Bee pollen also seems to have the ability to reduce prostatic inflammation that causes urinary tract blockage.

Capsaicin: hot on the cancer trail

Chilies may be the most popular spice in the world, but you need a hardy constitution and an iron stomach — or maybe you just need to be a bit of a masochist — to eat them every day. On the other hand, a capsaicin supplement may be helpful.

Capsaicin is the active ingredient that gives chilies their trademark hot-hot hotness. Capsaicin is also a hot supplement, most noteworthy for the well-documented pain relief it offers people with arthritis, but it is also a leading contender as a promising prostate protector.

In research at Cedars-Sinai Medical Center in Los Angeles, for example, capsaicin supplements caused death to 80 percent of cancer cells in test animals and tumors shrank to one-fifth of their size compared to animals that did not get capsaicin. The same study also found that capsaicin brought down PSA levels, which led the researchers to believe that capsaicin some day may play a role in helping to prevent disease recurrence in men treated for prostate cancer.

Though results of human studies are not yet available, dozens of animal and test-tube experiments have found that capsaicin has the ability to protect the prostate in multiple ways. It can help:

- induce death in cancer cells and slow tumor growth.

- lower PSA, a biomarker for prostate disease.

- slow cancer progression in tumors that do not respond well to hormone therapy.

- inhibit the production of dihydrotestosterone (DHT), the active form of the male hormone testosterone that is responsible for male sexuality and is also a possible factor in cancer growth.

- inhibit tumor necrosis factor (TNF), a Jeckyl-and-Hyde protein that plays a key role in triggering the inflammation associated with cancer.

Researchers at UCLA School of Medicine, who did many of these studies, called capsaicin effects on preventing and treating prostate cancer "profound." And researchers, reporting in the journal *Cancer Research*, found capsaicin a "potential target for the action of drugs in the management of prostate cancer" and its recurrence.

(Also see *Chilies*, page 249.)

Flaxseed oil: the fish oil alternative

Vegetarian? If fish doesn't cross your lips even as a supplement, then consider taking flaxseed oil. It offers your prostate everything fish oil does — plus one. In addition to omega-3 fatty acids, flaxseed oil contains a healthy dose of lignans, a type of phytoestrogen with powerful antioxidant qualities that work as a team to help keep prostate disease at bay.

In one study, reported in the *Journal of Medicinal Foods*, 87 men with BPH who took supplemental flaxseed oil every day for four months reported finding significant relief from lower urinary tract problems. The higher the dosage, the more their results improved on the International Prostate Symptom Score (IPSS), which measures the severity of BPH and its impact on quality of life. (You can find the IPSS on page 43).

In another study, 15 men who were scheduled to undergo a repeat prostate biopsy were instructed to follow a low-fat diet, consisting of no more than 20 percent of calories from fat, supplemented with flaxseed oil prior to the test. The diet resulted in "statistically significant decreases in PSA," according to the researchers from Duke University Medical Center. At a six-month follow-up, PSA was so low in two of the men that their planned biopsies were cancelled. The results, concluded the researchers, "suggest that a flaxseed-supplemented, fat-restricted diet may affect the biology of the prostate."

Adding flax to your food

Flaxseed is a type of grain with a nutty flavor. The seeds must be ground in order to digest them. Grinding, however, is messy and it makes the seeds highly perishable. As a result, many nutritionists recommend taking flaxseed in its purest form — as an oil straight from the bottle. To make it more palatable you can mix it in yogurt, smoothies, or protein shakes.

The oil is fragile and can turn rancid if not stored properly. It does not take well to heat, light, and oxygen, so it should be kept in an opaque bottle in the refrigerator. Buy oil that is cold pressed to help assure quality.

Caution: Consuming flax not only will reduce the circulation of DHT, the active form of testosterone, but may actually produce feminization with effects such as breast enlargement.

Put that 'B' back in the bottle

Don't bank your prostate health on taking a daily folic acid supplement in place of eating vitamin B-rich foods. It might leave you with serious regrets.

Initially, reports suggested that taking folic acid — the supplemental version of the B vitamin folate — might be protective against prostate cancer, an observation that came from looking at the cancer rates among different populations. The truth, it turns out, may be just the opposite.

A recent long-term population study concluded that folic acid supplements might increase the risk of prostate cancer. The study, which followed 643 men for 10 years, found that those who took folic acid supplements had a higher risk of getting prostate cancer compared to men taking a placebo.

Eating folate-rich foods, however, is still considered prostate-friendly. A study of 27,101 healthy male smokers found that high dietary levels of folate — but not from folate supplements — had a "significant protective effect" against prostate cancer.

Hops: brewing a secret nutrient

Someday when you raise a stein of beer and say, *Here's to your health!*, you may be talking about your prostate. Hops, best known as the agent that gives beer its bitter taste and aroma, is a medicinal herb that could some day play a role in the prevention and treatment of prostate disease.

It's not the medicinal herb per se that has attracted the attention of researchers but its most active ingredient, an antioxidant flavonoid called xanthohumol. As an antioxidant, scientists say it is stronger than vitamin E.

"We hope that one day we can demonstrate that xanthohumol prevents prostate cancer development, first in animal models and then in humans, but we are just at the beginning," said Clarissa Gerhauser, Ph.D., group leader of cancer chemoprevention in the Division of Epigenomics and Cancer Risk Factors at the German Cancer Research Center in Heidelberg, Germany.

Researchers are attracted to xanthohumol because lab studies show it can naturally stop the production of testosterone, which is associated with both the growth of the prostate that leads to BPH and the proliferation of prostate cells.

Since xanthohumol is only present in very small doses in regular beer, it would take an unhealthy amount of beer to get the same healing effect found in the lab. In addition, current xanthohumol supplements are not absorbed in the intestines — they are simply expelled as waste. For these reasons, researchers are working hard to develop a formula that can pass from your gastrointestinal tract into your blood. Keep your eyes peeled for a water-soluble liquid concentrate you can add to water or another beverage. It may be available soon.

Saw palmetto:
prostate protection, Southern style

If you have lots of LUTS — that's lower urinary tract symptoms — don't be too surprised if your doctor sends you to the health food store for some saw palmetto instead of giving you a prescription for medication. The herb is widely believed to be an effective natural remedy for relieving the symptoms of BPH. More than half the urologists in Germany swear by it and prefer it as a treatment to prescription drugs. Even Western medicine recognizes its effectiveness.

Saw palmetto is a small plant that grows in and around the Florida Everglades. Legend has it that the Seminole Indians who inhabited the region more than two centuries ago ate its seeds to help ease a puzzling problem — a sputtering and weak urine stream. As is well-know today, they were definitely on to something.

Saw palmetto works by inhibiting the enzyme that turns testosterone into dihydrotestosterone (DHT), thus stopping the abnormal proliferation of prostate cells and reducing swelling of the prostate — the same mechanisms by which the prescription prostate drug finasteride (Proscar) works. However, saw palmetto does the job in a different and, apparently, more effective way. Studies have found it is just as effective as finasteride — but with less of the numerous side effects, including face and breast swelling and sexual dysfunction, that are associated with prostate remedies that inhibit the action of testosterone.

Another study compared saw palmetto to tamsulosin (Flomax), a drug that helps improve urine flow, and found it worked even better — and without the side effects that can also interfere with your love life. This study, which included more than 800 men living in 11 European countries and lasted for one year, found that symptoms declined in both groups and PSA levels remained stable. However, prostate size diminished only in the group taking the herb and the men taking the drug reported difficulty maintaining an erection. In addition, saw palmetto worked faster. Men taking the herb reported improvement after only three months of treatment.

Finally, an analysis of 14 studies involving more than 14,000 men who used saw palmetto found that it brought "significant improvement" in peak urine flow rate and reduced the need to get up in the middle of the night to go to the bathroom. Also, it reduced their scores in the Chronic Prostatitis Symptom Index (CPSI) quality-of-life survey by a significant five points.

Unfortunately, saw palmetto, like other treatments that interfere with the action of testosterone, does not seem to improve mortality from prostate cancer.

Combination therapy for BPH

Sometimes good things come in bigger packages. Take the combination of bee pollen extract, saw palmetto, B-sitosterol, and vitamin E to reduce the chronic symptoms of BPH.

Each of these natural products has been shown to help decrease the symptoms of BPH, which led researchers from Georgetown University to suspect that combination therapy might work even better.

For the experiment they recruited 177 men with BPH and no evidence of cancer, who were being treated in three different urology centers around the country. The men received either the combination therapy or a placebo. Those taking the therapy showed a "markedly significant decrease in the severity" of sleep disturbances caused by the need to get up in the middle of the night to urinate compared to those taking the placebo. Daytime frequency also "lessened significantly."

Overall they found a "highly significant" difference in the symptom index score used to measure the severity of BPH.

Stinging nettle extract: the 'hurt' that heals

Stinging nettle is nothing you want to mess with if you find it in the woods, but men with BPH might want to wrap their arms around it when they see it in the bottle. Several studies show that the nonedible herb may be just as effective as the gold standard saw palmetto in reducing the symptoms of BPH. And, like saw palmetto, it has attracted big fans among European natural healers.

In one large study, researchers in Iran followed 558 men with BPH who were randomly given daily doses of either stinging nettle extract or a placebo. The researchers followed them for 18 months, routinely checking up on their symptoms. At the end of the study, 81 percent of the men taking the herb experienced significant relief in urinary symptoms compared to only 16 percent of the men taking the placebo. The researchers checked in with the men taking the herb after another year and a half. Only those who continued the therapy reported continued relief. The study was reported in the *Journal of Pharmacotherapy*.

Researchers believe that stinging nettle works the same way as saw palmetto — by inhibiting DHT, the substance in the male hormone testosterone that is suspected of causing the prostate to grow. This inhibition also reduces male sexuality as a side effect.

Herbal experts recommend drinking it as a tea.

Part 4

Resources

Support groups:
why they matter

Men can be reluctant givers when it comes to sharing and shedding emotion among strangers, but it's in your best interest to do the best you can to put your reluctance aside. Studies show that support groups have a profound positive impact on the overall well-being and longevity of their members. Studies also show that people who gain the most out of being part of a support group are men with prostate cancer.

Think about it. There is nothing to lose and a lot to gain. Support groups work so well because there are only two motives for joining — seeking help and helping others. They offer valuable insight into both the physical and emotional trials of your disease. They also offer something that you rarely find in many doctors — compassion.

Though each one operates in its own fashion, support groups have a common goal — to give and share information, offer encouragement and support, and be a forum for exchanging personal experiences and expressing opinions. Many groups are highly organized with monthly meetings, guest speakers, and panel discussions. Going to a support group is also a convenient way to find out about the quality of urologists, cancer specialists, and treatment centers in your area. It is not unusual to come across a member so absorbed in his illness that his self-learned expertise is on par with a doctor.

Spouses and significant others can get as much out of a support group as the men dealing with prostate disease or the unfortunate consequences of surgery. They, too, feel the emotional impact of their loved one's illness and often carry the burden in lonely silence. Support groups offer them the emotional support and the understanding hearts of other women in the same circumstances.

There is another way to share and get information about prostate problems. Studies have found that online support groups are just as beneficial to men with prostate disease, erectile dysfunction, and incontinence as face-to-face organizations.

Here is a list of some of the best-known support groups organized by the problems discussed in this book. At the end is a list of reliable organizations where you can find more information about your particular problem.

Benign prostatic hyperplasia support groups

Daily Strength

Daily Strength is an anonymous community of support groups for a variety of conditions.

Website: *www.dailystrength.org*

Web address to get to the enlarged prostate support group: *www.dailystrength.org/c/Enlarged-Prostate/support-group*

Drug Information Online

Drug Information Online offers support group questions and answers and a blog about prescription medications for BPH.

Website: *www.drugs.com*

To link to the BPH support group go to: *www.drugs.com/answers/support-group/benign-prostatic-hyperplasia-bph/*

Health Network

This interactive website offers an interactive support group for men with BPH to connect with doctors, experts, and other patients throughout the world.

Website: *www.healthnetwork.com*

To get information on the site's BPH support group go to: *www.medindia.net/healthnetwork/support-groups/benign-prostatic-hyperplasia.htm*

Inspire

Inspire offers support group memberships for a variety of health conditions. Men who join Inspire's BPH support group can connect with other people affected by the condition and let others know how they are doing.

Website: *www.inspire.com*

Web address to get you to the BPH support group: *www.inspire.com/conditions/benign-prostatic-hyperplasia-bph/*

Prostatitis support groups

Daily Strength

Daily Strength is an anonymous community of support groups for a variety of conditions.

Website: *www.dailystrength.org*

Web address to get you to the prostatitis support group: *www.dailystrength.org/c/Prostatitis/support-group*

iMedix.com

This online forum helps people with chronic disease find and share information and exchange personal experiences about their disease.

Website: *www.imedix.com*

Web address to get you to the prostatitis support group: *www.imedix.com/prostatitis*

MD Junction

MD Junction bills itself as "a community that is run by a community" and offers patient support groups for a variety of illnesses.

Website: *www.mdjunction.com*

Web address to get you to the prostatitis support group: *www.mdjunction.com/prostatitis*

Prostate cancer support groups

Daily Strength

Daily Strength is an anonymous community of support groups for a variety of conditions.

Website: *www.dailystrength.org*

Web address to get you to the prostate cancer support group: *www.dailystrength.org/c/Prostate-Cancer/support-group*

Man to Man

The American Cancer Society is the co-sponsor of this community-based support group for men with prostate cancer and their families. Meetings are held monthly at local centers around the country.

Website: *www.cancer.org*

Web address to find a group in your community: *www.cancer.org/treatment/supportprogramsservices/man toman*

Phone: 800-227-2345

Malecare, Inc.

Live online support groups of patients and doctors who write weekly updates on treatments and their side effects.

Website: *www.malecare.org*

MD Junction

MD Junction bills itself as "a community that is run by a community" and offers patient support groups for a variety of illnesses.

Website: *www.mdjunction.com*

Web address to get you to the prostate cancer support group: *www.mdjunction.com/prostate-cancer*

PSA Rising

This cancer survivors support network offers information on finding a local support group near you.

Website: *www.psa-rising.com*

To link directly to support group information, go to: *www.psa-rising.com/caplinks/support.htm*

Support Groups.com

This is a site of interactive support groups for a variety of illnesses.

Website: *www.supportgroups.com*

To link directly to a prostate cancer support group, go to: *www.prostate-cancer.supportgroups.com/*

Women Against Prostate Cancer

This is a nationwide advocacy organization that provides support to the millions of women affected by prostate cancer.

Website: *www.womenagainstprostatecancer.org*

Us TOO International, Inc.

This grassroots organization was started in 1990 by prostate cancer survivors to help educate and offer support to men with the disease. There are more than 300 support groups nation-wide. You can find one closest to you by going to their website.

Website: *www.ustoo.org*

Incontinence support groups

Continence Restored, Inc.

This organization, which has no website, offers information and telephone support to people with incontinence.

Phone: 203-348-0601 or 914-285-1470

Daily Strength

Daily Strength is an anonymous community of support groups for a variety of conditions.

Website: *www.dailystrength.org*

Web address to get you to the incontinence support group: *www.dailystrength.org/c/Urinary-Incontinence/support-group*

MD Junction

MD Junction bills itself as "a community that is run by a community" and offers patient support groups for a variety of illnesses.

Website: *www.mdjunction.com*

Web address to get you to the incontinence support group: *www.mdjunction.com/urinary-incontinence*

National Association for Continence

This organization is a telephone support network dedicated to improving the quality of life for people with incontinence. It also offers a newsletter, regional conferences, information, and referrals.

Website: *www.nafc.org*

Phone: 800-252-337

Erectile dysfunction support groups

Daily Strength

Daily Strength is an anonymous community of support groups for a variety of conditions.

Website: *www.dailystrength.org*

Web address to get you to the support group: *www.dailystrength.org/c/Impotence-Erectile-Dysfunction/ support-group*

ErectileDysfunctionConnection.com

This organization, which is affiliated with healthcentral.com, can put you in touch with someone you can talk to about erectile dysfunction.

Website: *www.healthcentral.com*

Web address to get you to the Erectile Dysfunction Connection: *www.healthcentral.com/erectile-dysfunction/*

MD Junction

MD Junction bills itself as "a community that is run by a community" and offers patient support groups for a variety of illnesses.

Website: *www.mdjunction.com*

Web address to get you to the erectile dysfunction support group: *www.mdjunction.com/erectile-dysfunction*

Information sources

American Cancer Society

The American Cancer Society offers specific, comprehensive information on all types of cancer.

Website: *www.cancer.org*

To link directly to prostate cancer go to: *www.cancer.org/cancer/prostatecancer/index*

Email: info@cancerrecovery.org

Phone: 800-227-2345

Write: 250 Williams St., N.W., Atlanta, GA 30303

American Urological Association

The AUA offers patient information on prostate cancer and incontinence.

Website: *www.urologyhealth.org*

Email: auafoundation@auafoundation.org

Phone: 800-828-7866

Write: 1000 Corporate Blvd., Linthicum, MD 21090

Foundation for Cancer Research and Wellness

This is an advocacy organization for less toxic and minimally invasive prevention and survival techniques for people with cancer.

Website: *www.cancerresearchandwellness.org*

Phone: 800-238-6479

Write: P.O. Box 1, Hershey, PA 17033

Prostate Cancer Foundation

This is a philanthropic organization with a mission to organize and fund research to find a cure for prostate cancer. It offers patient information on all aspects of the disease.

Website: *www.pcf.org*

Email: info@pcf.org

Phone: 800-757-2873

Write: 1250 Fourth Street, Santa Monica, CA 90401

Prostate Cancer Research Institute

This organization provides up-to-date information on the latest findings in prostate research. It also offers a free newsletter called *Insights*.

Website: *www.prostate-cancer.org*

Email: info@pcri.org or help@pcri.org

Phone: 800-641-7274

Write: 5777 W. Century Blvd., Suite 800, Los Angeles, CA 90045

Prostatitis Foundation

The Prostatitis Foundation is dedicated to collecting data, publishing research, and providing information to men with the disease.

Website: *www.prostatitis.org*

Phone: 888-891-4200

Write: 1063 30th St., Box 8, Smithshire, IL 61478

The Prostate Net

The organization offers men with prostate cancer and their families the support and tools to navigate their treatment options.

Website: *www.prostate-online.org*

Email: support@prostatenet.org

Phone: 888-477-6763

Write: P.O. Box 2192, Secaucus, NJ 07096-2192

Simon Foundation for Continence

This organization is dedicated to removing the stigma of incontinence and offers help and support for people with the condition.

Website: *www.simonfoundation.org*

Email: webmaster@simonfoundation.org

Phone: 800-237-4666

Write: P.O. Box 815, Wilmette, IL 60091

And the answers are ...

These are the correct answers to the quiz on page 28:

1. 1 to 5 percent will die of prostate cancer.

2. 15 to 25 percent will be diagnosed as having prostate cancer at some time in their lives.

3. 20 to 40 percent of the time it does turn out to be cancer.

America's top treatment centers for prostate disease

These hospitals and medical centers were ranked as tops in the nation for patient care and treatment by *U.S. News and World Report*.

Ranking	Cancer	Urology
1	University of Texas MD Anderson Cancer Center★ Houston, TX	Johns Hopkins Hospital★ Baltimore, MD
2	Memorial Sloan-Kettering Cancer Center★ New York, NY	Cleveland Clinic★ Cleveland, OH
3	Johns Hopkins Hospital★ Baltimore, MD	Mayo Clinic★ Rochester, MN
4	Mayo Clinic★ Rochester, MN	Ronald Reagan UCLA Medical Center★ Los Angeles, CA
5	Dana-Farber/Brigham and Women's Cancer Cancer Center★ Boston, MA	Memorial Sloan-Kettering Cancer Center★ New York, NY

Ranking	Cancer	Urology
6	University of Washington Medical Center Seattle, WA	University of California, San Francisco Medical Center★ San Francisco, CA
7	Massachusetts General Hospital★ Boston, MA	New York-Presbyterian University Hospital of Columbia and Cornell★ New York, NY
8	University of California, San Francisco Medical Center★ San Francisco, CA	Duke University Medical Center★ Durham, NC
9	Cleveland Clinic★ Cleveland, OH	Vanderbilt University Medical Center Nashville, TN
10	Ronald Reagan UCLA Medical Center★ Los Angeles, CA	University of Texas MD Anderson Cancer Center★ Houston, TX
11	Duke University Medical Center★ Durham, NC	Massachusetts General Hospital★ Boston, MA
12	Stanford Hospital and Clinics★ Palo Alto, CA	University of Texas Southwestern Medical Center Dallas, TX
13	University of Michigan Hospitals and Health Centers★ Ann Arbor, MI	Hospital of the University of Pennsylvania★ Philadelphia, PA
14	University of Chicago Medical Center Chicago, IL	Indiana University Health Indianapolis, IN
15	Hospital of the University of Pennsylvania★ Philadelphia, PA	University of Michigan Hospitals and Health Centers★ Ann Arbor, MI

Ranking	Cancer	Urology
16	Barnes-Jewish Hospital/ Washington University ★ Saint Louis, MO	Stanford Hospital and Clinics ★ Palo Alto, CA
17	City of Hope Duarte, CA	Barnes-Jewish Hospital/ Washington University ★ Saint Louis, MO
18	Moffitt Cancer Center Tampa, FL	USC University Hospital Los Angeles, CA
19	New York-Presbyterian University Hospital of Columbia and Cornell ★ New York, NY	Dana-Farber/Brigham and Women's Hospital ★ Boston, MA
20	Ohio State University James Cancer Hospital Columbus, OH	Northwestern Memorial Hospital ★ Chicago, IL
21	Northwestern Memorial Hospital ★ Chicago, IL	University of Iowa Hospitals and Clinics Iowa City, IA
22	University of Maryland Medical Center Baltimore, MD	Lahey Clinic Burlington, MA
23	University of Minnesota Medical Center Minneapolis, MN	Methodist Hospital Houston, TX
24	Yale-New Haven Hospital New Haven, CT	Shands at the University of Florida Gainesville, FL
25	NYU Langone Medical Center ★ New York, NY	NYU Langone Medical Center ★ New York, NY

★ = ranked as one of the best 25 hospitals for both urology and cancer
Adapted from U.S. News Best Hospitals 2011-12

The treatment with the best overall outcome for many cases of prostate cancer may be brachytherapy. Here are 21 doctors that, according to *U.S. News and World Report* and the independent healthcare rating firm, Castle Connolly Medical Ltd., are top in the specialized field of brachytherapy. In fact, these physicians are considered among the top 1 percent in the nation in brachytherapy.

These doctors were nominated for this selection by their peers, and their education, training, hospital appointments, history, and much more, were screened by the Castle Connolly research team. Many are also affiliated with a top-ranking cancer or urology treatment facility.

Doctors with expertise in brachytherapy	Admitting hospital
Mitchell S. Anscher, MD	Virginia Commonwealth University Medical Center
Jonathan J. Beitler, MD	Emory University Hospital
Jay P. Ciezki, MD	Cleveland Clinic
Anthony D'Amico, MD/PhD	Dana-Farber/Brigham and Women's Cancer Center
Ronald D. Ennis, MD	Beth Israel Medical Center
Glen Gejerman, MD	Hackensack University Medical Center
Gordon L. Grado, MD	Scottsdale Healthcare Shea Medical Center
Louis B. Harrison, MD	Beth Israel Medical Center
Randal H. Henderson, MD	Shands at the University of Florida
Eric Horwitz, MD	Fox Chase Cancer Center
Anuja Jhingran, MD	University of Texas MD Anderson Cancer Center

Doctors with expertise in brachytherapy	Admitting hospital
Irving Kaplan, MD	Beth Israel Deaconess Medical Center
Wu-Jin Koh, MD	University of Washington Medical Center
Mahesh Kudrimoti, MD	University of Kentucky Albert B. Chandler Hospital
W. Robert Lee, MD	Duke University Medical Center
Arnold Malcolm, MD	Vanderbilt University Medical Center
Dattatreyudu Nori, MD	New York-Presbyterian University Hospital of Columbia and Cornell
Leonard M. Toonkel, MD	Mount Sinai Medical Center
Michael J. Zelefsky, MD	Memorial Sloan-Kettering Cancer Center
Frank A. Vicini, MD	Beaumont Hospital
Srinivasan Vijayakumar, MD	University of Mississippi Health Care

Prostate terminology defined

A

Active surveillance — Actively monitoring low- and sometimes intermediate-risk prostate cancer by having regular physicals, PSA tests, and perhaps biopsies or other tests, but otherwise delaying treatment until or if the cancer progresses to a stage where treatment is the better option.

Acute bacterial prostatitis — A rare condition that involves sudden, sometimes severe, inflammation or infection of the prostate. Symptoms include fever and burning during urination. Generally responds quickly to antibiotics.

Acute urinary retention — Condition that requires immediate medical attention, occurring when the urethra is squeezed so tightly by the prostate that it becomes impossible to urinate. Things that can trigger urinary retention include delaying urination, urinary tract infection, alcohol intake, antidepressants, decongestants, tranquilizers, cold temperatures, and being still for long periods of time.

Alpha blockers — The same medicine used to treat high blood pressure that can relieve BPH and incontinence symptoms in men with an enlarged prostate. Relaxes the smooth muscles that are squeezing the urethra, making it harder for urine to get through.

Androgen-dependent cells — Prostate cancer cells that need androgen hormones to grow. Hormone therapy will control these kinds of cells.

Androgen deprivation therapy — A treatment option that suppresses the production of the male hormone testosterone, generally used for men with advanced, recurring cancer.

Androgen-independent cells — Prostate cancer cells that don't need androgen hormones to grow. No treatments, including hormone therapy, will control these kinds of cells.

Androgens — Male hormones.

Angiogenesis — The body's process of forming new blood vessels.

Anticholinergic drugs — A class of drugs that suppresses bladder contractions.

Artificial sphincter — A three-part device that is surgically implanted near the bladder to control incontinence.

Asymptomatic — Experiencing no sign of symptoms.

Atherosclerosis — A condition in which fatty deposits build up in your blood vessels, restricting blood flow. A common cause of impotence, especially in older men.

B

Benign — Noncancerous.

Benign prostatic hyperplasia (BPH) — A noncancerous enlargement of the prostate gland that commonly affects half the men over age 60.

Extra tissue grows inside the prostate and presses on the urethra. This prevents your bladder from being emptied completely and leads to annoying symptoms like dribbling, a slow stream, and frequent urination.

Beta blockers — A drug option for men who need prostate surgery but have heart disease or are at risk of heart disease.

Biochemical failure — Returning prostate cancer detected by a rising PSA.

Biofeedback — Learning to control various automatic body functions such as heart rate, blood pressure, and temperature. Leads are placed on the body that are connected to a device which emits visual and sound clues when the desired change occurs. By observing these signals, the person can learn to produce the desired change voluntarily. Incontinence can be treated with this technique.

Biopsy — Inserting a small needle through the rectum and up into the prostate to remove tissue samples. A pathologist will examine this tissue and look for cancer cells.

Bladder — A muscular pouch that temporarily stores urine until it can be excreted from your body.

Bladder training — A technique for controlling incontinence. It teaches you to control your urges and gradually go longer and longer before urinating.

Brachytherapy — A type of radiation used to treat prostate cancer in which 80 to 120 radioactive seeds are inserted into the prostate. The seeds are left in place permanently and continue to emit low levels of radiation for a few months.

C

Castrate range — The level of testosterone seen in men who have had their testicles removed.

Castration — Surgical removal of the testicles.

Catheter — A slender, hollow tube used especially for draining urine from the bladder.

Central zone — The second-largest part of the prostate.

Chemical castration — The use of drugs to lower testosterone.

Chemotherapy — Special cell-killing drugs used to treat cancer.

Chronic bacterial prostatitis — A fairly rare condition that involves infection plus inflammation of the prostate. Although antibiotics can help, it usually takes much longer to clear up this infection than acute bacterial prostatitis. This condition also appears to be linked with repeated urinary tract infections (UTIs).

Chronic pelvic pain syndrome — The new term for nonbacterial prostatitis and prostatodynia.

Clinical stage — The stage your doctor believes your cancer to be in. He bases his estimation on the results of a variety of tests, which often include the DRE, PSA screening, TRUS, and a biopsy.

Clinical trial — Researchers use clinical trials to find out if promising new treatment methods really work. If you participate in one of these treatment studies, you will be given the new treatment — or possibly a placebo — and carefully watched. All your reactions will be written down and compared with others.

Cryosurgery — Also called cryosurgical ablation of the prostate (CSAP) or cryotherapy, this "ice cube" surgery attempts to eliminate cancer by freezing the cells to death.

D

Digital rectal exam (DRE) — To check your prostate, your doctor will insert a gloved, lubricated finger into your rectum and press down. He will try to determine if your prostate has any hard lumps, which may suggest cancer, or if any areas feel tender and soft, which may indicate infection. A healthy prostate feels firm and elastic to the touch.

Dihydrotestosterone (DHT) — What testosterone is converted to once it reaches the prostate. This is the active form of testosterone in the prostate. The 5-alpha reductase enzymes are responsible for this conversion.

E

Ejaculation — The exit of semen from the body that normally occurs during sexual climax.

Ejaculatory duct — The channel formed by the vas deferens and the seminal vesicle. It joins the prostatic urethra.

Erectile dysfunction — Consistently unable to become erect or stay erect long enough to have intercourse.

Estrogen — Female hormone that can stop testosterone from being produced by the testicles.

External beam radiation — A type of radiation therapy that bombards the general vicinity of the prostate in order to destroy the cancer cells.

External urethral sphincter — The muscle men use to control the release of urine.

F

Finasteride — One of the most prescribed medications for prostate problems. It works by slowing tissue growth and sometimes even shrinking your prostate to unblock your urethra. In addition, it blocks the conversion of testosterone to dihydrotestosterone, which tends to promote prostate enlargement. May help prevent prostate cancer. It is also used to treat cases of advanced prostate cancer.

G

Gleason grade / Gleason score — The most widely accepted cancer grading system. It is based on how cancer looks under the microscope. Cancers are classified as well-differentiated, moderately differentiated, or poorly differentiated. Poorly differentiated cancers are considered the most aggressive, which means the cancer is more likely to progress and spread throughout the body.

H

High intensity focused ultrasound (HIFU) — Uses highly controlled and concentrated ultrasound energy like a scalpel to treat BPH. This method focuses energy directly on the area that needs to be destroyed, sparing the surrounding healthy tissue. However, it usually causes temporary urinary retention and blood in the semen. Long-term effects are not known, and researchers suspect it may not be effective in men with large prostate glands.

Hormone therapy — Lowers male hormone levels to shrink or slow the progression of prostate cancer. Usually causes a loss of sexual desire and impotence.

I

Impotence — The inability to experience sexual intercourse, especially because of an inability to have an erection.

Incontinence — Inability to control the flow of urine.

Interstitial Laser Coagulation of the Prostate (ILCP) — Ultrasound used to direct placement of laser fibers.

Interstitial radiation — See Brachytherapy.

K

Kegel exercises — Exercises to strengthen and tone the muscles that control urination. Many doctors recommend you begin these immediately after a radical prostatectomy. These exercises can also help treat impotence.

Kidneys — Where urine formation begins. Your body breaks down the food you eat into chemical byproducts, which are transported by your bloodstream to the kidneys. The kidneys then filter your blood to collect the waste and excess water, forming urine.

L

Luteinizing hormone (LH) — A hormone produced by the pituitary gland. LH is responsible for telling the Leydig cells in your prostate to release testosterone into your bloodstream.

Luteinizing hormone-releasing hormone (LHRH) antagonists — Drugs that prevent the release of or interfere with the action of male hormones. A commonly used hormone therapy for prostate cancer, LHRH antagonists shut off the supply of testosterone from the testicles by blocking the pituitary's production of LH. Sometimes referred to as medical orchiectomy.

Lycopene — A carotenoid associated with a reduced risk of prostate cancer. The substance in tomatoes that gives them their red color. Also found in watermelon, pink grapefruit, guava, papaya, apricots, and rose hips.

M

Mixed incontinence — A combination of incontinence symptoms. For men with an enlarged prostate, the most common combination is urge incontinence and overflow incontinence.

N

Neoadjuvant hormone therapy — Drugs to shut down the production of testosterone and prevent potential cancer spread. Generally, neoadjuvant hormone therapy is reserved for men with cancer that has spread into tissue right outside the prostate.

Nerve-sparing prostatectomy — Surgical technique that cuts close to the prostate, taking care to spare nearby nerves. This technique reduces the risk of impotence.

Nonbacterial prostatitis (NBP) — The most common type of prostatitis with inflammation in the prostate but no infection and no sign of bacteria. May or may not respond to antibiotics.

O

Oncologist — Doctor specially trained to diagnose and treat cancer.

Open prostatectomy — A type of surgery usually reserved for men who have very large prostates that make performing TURP or TUIP unsafe. It involves making an incision in the lower part of the stomach area and removing the prostate through the bladder or cutting directly into the prostate itself.

Orchiectomy — Surgical removal of the testicles.

Overflow incontinence — Occurs when an enlarged prostate presses against the urethra, blocking the flow of urine out of your body. Your bladder becomes too full, and small amounts of urine dribble out uncontrollably.

P

Partin tables — Named after the Johns Hopkins doctor who created them, these tables combine information from your PSA level, your Gleason score, and your estimated clinical stage (based on the TNM system) to determine the pathological stage of your cancer. They tell you the likelihood that the cancer is still confined to your prostate or has spread beyond. Helpful for choosing a treatment strategy.

Pathological stage — The stage of your cancer, based on a pathologist's examination of actual prostate tissue or based on data from the Partin tables.

Pathologist — A doctor who specializes in diagnosing abnormal changes in tissue samples.

Penile clamp — A device used to control incontinence by squeezing the shaft of the penis so that no urine can flow through.

Penile cuff — A comfortable inflatable band that does much the same thing as the penile clamp.

Penile implants — In cases of impotence, a semirigid device can be surgically inserted into your penis to produce either a permanent erection or an erection that can be controlled by using a pump. Several different types of implants are available, ranging from a simple malleable rod to sophisticated hydraulic pump systems.

Perineal radical prostatectomy — In this approach, the surgeon goes through the perineal region to reach the prostate. This is generally considered to be a less strenuous surgery so it may be used in older men or in men with poorer health who may have higher risks of complications and who would not be troubled by consequent erectile dysfunction. Used only for prostate cancer.

Perineum — The area between the penis and the anus.

Peripheral zone — The area making up the majority of the prostate.

Pressure flow studies — This test measures the pressure in your bladder as you urinate. That number is then compared to the speed of your urine stream. Some doctors feel this test is the best way to find out how much your ability to urinate is affected. A small tube called a catheter is inserted into your penis, through the urethra, and into your bladder. This study will confirm whether or not you will benefit from surgery.

Priapism — Prolonged erection that can cause permanent damage to your penis.

Prostascint — This test can accurately detect cancer spread outside the prostate. A harmless radioactive particle is injected, which then reveals the exact location of all the cancer.

Prostate gland — The part-muscle, part-gland structure that produces nutrient-rich secretions that combine with sperm to make semen.

Prostate massage — Rubbing the prostate to help drain it and increase blood flow to it.

Prostate-specific antigen (PSA) — PSA is a protein that is secreted into your prostatic ducts during ejaculation. The main purpose of PSA is to liquefy semen after ejaculation so sperm may be released on their journey to find an available egg to fertilize. Since the early 1990s, doctors have used the measurement of PSA levels to test for possible prostate cancer.

Prostate-specific antigen (PSA) test — Measures your levels of PSA. High PSA levels signal you have a problem with your prostate.

Your doctor may use this test to confirm his suspicions of either BPH or prostate cancer.

Prostate stones — Similar to stones found in the gallbladder or kidneys, these are one of the main causes of a prostate infection that fails to respond to treatment. Prostate stones are normally harmless unless they harbor bacteria. Then, they serve as a breeding ground for repeated infections.

Prostatectomy — Prostate surgery. A prostatectomy for BPH removes all the tissue inside the prostate, leaving only the prostatic capsule. A radical prostatectomy for prostate cancer removes the entire prostate.

Prostatic — Having to do with the prostate gland.

Prostatic capsule — The muscular tissue enclosing the entire prostate.

Prostatic fluid — The thin liquid secreted by the prostate that combines with sperm to make semen.

Prostatic intraepithelial neoplasia (PIN) — Abnormal, benign lesions that have a strong link to cancer. If your biopsy points out PIN, you should have another one. About half the time another biopsy will find cancer.

Prostatic urethra — The part of the urethra completely encircled by the prostate gland.

Prostatitis — An inflamed prostate gland, which may or may not be infected. Prostatitis is a general term that includes infections, inflammation, and nonbacterial conditions of the prostate. There are three types of prostatitis: acute bacterial prostatitis, chronic bacterial prostatitis, and chronic nonbacterial prostatitis, by far the most common type.

PSA density (PSAD) — This measurement is useful for distinguishing men with BPH from men with prostate cancer. It is determined by dividing your PSA number by the volume of your prostate. The higher your PSA density, the greater your risk of cancer.

PSA velocity (PSAV) — Also known as serial PSA testing, the velocity measures annual changes in PSA levels.

Pulmonary embolism — A blood clot that plugs the arteries supplying blood to the lungs. One of the possible complications of prostate surgery, especially an open prostatectomy.

R

Radiation therapy (radiotherapy) — The use of high-energy waves to stop the progress of prostate cancer by interfering with cancer cell reproduction. Radiation is a good option when the cancer has penetrated the prostate capsule but has only spread to surrounding tissue.

Radical prostatectomy — Surgical procedure that removes the entire prostate gland.

Residual urine test — This procedure is designed to show if the bladder empties normally or not. A catheter is inserted into the bladder to empty and measure any remaining urine.

Retrograde ejaculation — When semen backs up into the bladder instead of being forced out through the penis. This renders most men infertile but should not interfere with the sensation of orgasm. Also called "dry ejaculation."

Retropubic prostatectomy — The most common type of radical prostatectomy. The surgeon cuts into the lower section of your abdominal area behind the pubic bone to get to your prostate. This approach may be used for either open prostatectomy (for BPH) or radical prostatectomy (for prostate cancer).

S

Scrotum — The sac of skin that contains the testicles.

Semen — The fluid containing sperm which comes out of the penis during sexual excitement.

Seminal vesicles — Small sacs connected to the vas deferens that produce nutrient-rich secretions that combine with sperm to make semen.

Sperm — A reproductive cell capable of fertilizing a woman's egg, which, if timing is right and conditions are good, may eventually develop into a baby.

Sphincter — A ring-shaped muscle that surrounds various openings in the body and can control its opening and closing by contracting or expanding.

Staging — A way of categorizing the different levels of cancer development.

Stress incontinence — Urine leakage triggered by coughing, sneezing, or straining. This usually happens when the muscle that controls urine flow, the bladder sphincter, becomes weak.

Suprapubic prostatectomy — A prostatectomy where the surgeon goes through your bladder to reach your prostate. This approach is only used for BPH.

T

Testicles — The two oval glands suspended in the scrotum that make sperm and testosterone.

Testosterone — A male steroid sex hormone, produced in the testicles and adrenal glands. Affects the growth of prostate tissue and male sexuality.

Timed voiding — A set schedule for urination that keeps your bladder emptied regularly and cuts the risk of involuntary leakage.

Total incontinence — A complete inability to control the release of urine.

Transcutaneous electrical nerve stimulation (TENS) — A pain relief option using mild electrical stimulation on your skin. This system provides nondrug relief by interfering with pain's pathway to your brain.

Transition zone — The smallest area of the prostate, making up only 5 to 10 percent of the entire gland.

Transrectal ultrasonography (TRUS) — During this procedure, a probe is inserted about 3 to 4 inches into your rectum. The probe makes images of your prostate and surrounding tissues as it is being removed. A urologist will use TRUS to determine the size of your prostate and identify areas that may be cancerous. If your doctor decides a biopsy is needed, he will use TRUS to help him guide the biopsy needle.

Transurethral incision of the prostate (TUIP) — An endoscopic surgical procedure limited to men with smaller prostates in which an instrument is passed through the urethra to make one or two cuts in the prostate and prostate capsule, reducing constriction of the urethra. This procedure can be done on an outpatient basis.

Transurethral microwave thermotherapy (TUMT) — An experimental procedure that involves sending computer-regulated microwave heat through a catheter to selected portions of the prostate to destroy excess prostate tissue. Because of the device's design, it can only be used in men with medium-sized prostates. Also, it may take six weeks to three months for changes to become significantly noticeable.

Transurethral needle ablation (TUNA) — A type of heat therapy that uses radio frequency energy to destroy excess prostate tissue. TUNA seems to work best in men who have slight obstructions.

Transurethral resection of the prostate (TUR or TURP) — Surgical removal of the prostate's inner portion by an endoscopic approach through the urethra, with no external incision. This is the most common treatment for symptomatic BPH and usually requires a hospital stay.

Transurethral vaporization of the prostate (TVP) — This procedure is similar to TURP, but instead of cutting away excess tissue, an electric current vaporizes the extra tissue. TVP involves a shorter hospital stay and perhaps less risk of bleeding, incontinence, or narrowing of the urethra.

Tumor, Node, Metastasis (TNM) system — A system for staging cancer. T indicates the size and spread of cancer within and near the prostate; N indicates if and where the cancer has spread to the lymph nodes; M indicates that cancer has spread to other organs and sites in the body.

U

Urethra — The tube that carries urine from the bladder through the penis and out of the body. It also carries semen from the prostatic urethra out of the body.

Urethral stricture — A problem that occurs when scar tissue from an injury or untreated infection in the urethra shrinks, causing the urethra to narrow and sometimes become shorter. This makes it difficult and painful to urinate or ejaculate. Surgery is often necessary to correct this problem.

Urethritis — An inflammation of the urethra. It may be caused by an infection, an irritation, or a minor injury.

Urge incontinence — Difficulty controlling urination possibly caused by a prostate infection or a prostatectomy. You feel the sudden need to urinate, but can't reach the bathroom in time.

Urinary retention — Incomplete emptying of the bladder.

Urinary (urethral) sphincter — The muscle that controls urine flow.

Uroflowmetry — Another name for the uroflow test. Simple and painless, all you need is a full bladder. You urinate into a special toilet, which measures how much urine you pass and records the speed of your urine stream.

Urologist — A doctor who specializes in treating disorders of the urinary system and male reproductive system.

V

Vacuum pump — This nonsurgical option for treating impotence uses a vacuum to pull blood into the penis. Once fully erect, a rubber ring is placed at the base of the penis to retain the blood until intercourse is completed.

Vas deferens — The system of tubes that conveys the sperm from the testicles to the penis. Also called ductus deferens.

Vasectomy — A form of male birth control which either ties or removes the vas deferens so that sperm cannot pass through.

Visualization — A technique to help control body processes by using a picture in your mind. You can learn different ways to soothe, heal, calm, or control your body.

Volume monitors — Specialized nerves in the trigone (base of bladder) and bladder wall that monitor the amount of urine in the bladder. Once enough liquid has collected, they signal the brain that the bladder needs to be emptied.

W

Watchful waiting — In prostate cancer, forgoing treatment because the prognosis for the disease does not look good, whether treated or not.

Index

A

Abdominal fat 223-224
Active surveillance. *See also*
  Watchful waiting
  cancer risk and 99
  definition of 12
  overview 164
  prostate cancer and 18, 111-
    115, 158
  weight and 222
Acupuncture 78-79
Acute bacterial prostatitis. *See*
  Prostatitis
Acute urinary retention 41
African plum extract 292
Age
  BPH and 39
  impotence and 201
  prostate cancer and 89
  PSA levels and 92
Aged garlic extract (AGE) 316
Alcohol
  BPH and 227
  gallic acid in 302
  impotence and 199
  incontinence and 187
  prostate cancer and 227
  resveratrol in 257, 297
Alfuzosin (Uroxatral) 52, 56
Alliums 242-244
Alpha blockers
  for BPH 56-57
  for prostatitis 77, 84
  PDE5 inhibitors and 204
Alpha-tocopherol 308
Alprostadil (Caverject) 207
American Cancer Society 339

American Urological
  Association 339
Anardana 265
AndroGel 145, 210
Androgen deprivation therapy
  140-147, 164
Androgen suppressants 53-54
Angiogenesis 236
Anthocyanins
  in apples 246
  in berries 247
  in cranberries 253
  in pomegranate 264
Anti-inflammatories 17, 77
Antiandrogen receptors 147
Anticoagulants 285
Antihistamines and BPH 48
Apoptosis 236
Apples 246
Apriso. *See* Mesalamine
Aredia. *See* Bisphosphonate
  pamidronate
Artificial light and prostate
  cancer 228
Artificial urinary sphincter 192-
  193
Aspirin 284-285
Atherosclerosis. *See* Heart disease
Avanafil 204
Aventyl. *See* Nortriptyline
Avodart. *See* Dutasteride
Azulfidine. *See* Sulfasalazine

B

Bee pollen extract 322-323

Benign prostatic hyperplasia.
See BPH (benign prostatic
hyperplasia)
Berries 246-247
Beta carotene 249, 310-311
Beta-sitosterol 302-303
Bicalutamide (Casodex) 147, 321
Bicycling 51, 80
Bilateral orchiectomy 140
Biochemical failure 157
Biofeedback 77-78, 189-190
Biopsy
    after PSA test 25
    overview 96-97
    results 98
    risks 98-99
    variables to consider 95
Bisphosphonate pamidronate
    (Aredia) 145
Black cohosh 306-307
Black cumin seeds 303-304
Blackberries 247
Bladder
    anatomy of 35
    incomplete emptying 41
Bladder cancer 42
Bladder outlet obstruction
    (BOO) 42, 46
Bladder pacemaker 192
Bladder stones 42
Bladder training 188
Blood sugar. See Diabetes
Blueberries 247
Body mass index (BMI) 222-223
Bone scan 104-105
Boron 267
Botox (Botulinum toxin type A)
    85
BPH (benign prostatic hyperpla-
    sia)
    abdominal fat and 223-224

age and 39
alcohol and 227
Botox for 85
definition of 16, 38
diagnosing 43-46
diet and 49-50, 233-279
exercise and 225-227
hair loss and 55-56
herbal remedies for 51
hormones and 38
Kegel exercises for 50-51
medications and 48
medications for 53-58
PDE5 inhibitors and 204
race and 39
retrograde ejaculation and 58
saturated fat and 238-239
sexual function and 52
stress and 51
support groups 333-334
surgery for 58-70
symptoms 38, 39
top-ranked hospitals for 342-
    344
treatment options 46-70
weight and 221-222
Brachytherapy 135-139
    overview 165
    risks 154
    top doctors for 345
Broccoli 248
Brussels sprouts 248

C

Cabbage 248
Caffeine
    BPH and 49
    incontinence and 187
    prostatitis and 84

Calcium 287
Canola oil 248
Capsaicin
    food sources 249-251
    supplemental 323-324
Carbohydrates 240, 277-278. *See also* Glycemic index
Cardura. *See* Doxazosin
Casodex. *See* Bicalutamide
Castration
    chemical 142
    surgical 140, 148
Catheterization 41
Cauliflower 248
Caverject. *See* Alprostadil
Celexa. *See* Citalopram
Central zone of the prostate gland 35
Cernilton 320
Cernitin 322
Chemotherapy 159
Chilies 249-251
Chlor Trimeton. *See* Pseudoephedrine
Cholesterol
    dietary 240-241
    hormone therapy and 141
Chronic bacterial prostatitis. *See* Prostatitis
Chronic Prostatitis Symptom Index (CPSI) 72-75
Cialis. *See* Tadalafil
Cipro. *See* Ciprofloxacin
Ciprofloxacin (Cipro) 76, 252
Circadian rhythm 228-230
Citalopram (Celexa) 77
Citrus fruits 251-252
Clinical trials 153
Clinical tumor grade 102
Collagen injections 191

Collard greens 249
Conference of Active Surveillance 13
Conjugated linoleic acid (CLA) 312-314
Cooking method 271. *See also* Grilling
Cooled thermo therapy 65-66
CPSI (Chronic Prostatitis Symptom Index) 72-75
Cranberries 247, 252-253
Cretan Diet 219-220
Cruciferous vegetables 247-249
Cryoablation surgery (cryotherapy) 149-151, 154, 166
Curcumin 290-292
Curry powder 292
Cymbalta. *See* Duloxetin
Cystometry 45

D

Da Vinci Surgical System 127-129
Daidzein 270, 318
Dairy foods
    calcium and 287
    CLA in 313
    prostate cancer and 239
Decongestants and BPH 44, 48
Degarelix (Firmagon) 147
Deltasone. *See* Prednisone
Depression
    impotence and 200
    prostatitis and 77
Detrol. *See* Tolterodine tartrate
Diabetes
    hormone therapy and 141, 142
    impotence and 200
    prostate cancer and 279
Diallyl disulfide (DADS) 316

Diet
  alliums 242-244
  apples 246
  berries 246-247
  BPH and 49-50
  canola oil 248
  carbohydrates 240
  chilies 249-251
  cholesterol 240-241
  citrus fruits 251-252
  cranberries 252-253
  Cretan Diet 219-220
  cruciferous vegetables 247-249
  dairy 239
  fish 253-257
  garlic 244
  grapes 257-258
  green tea 258-259
  incontinence and 187-188
  licorice 259-260
  low-fat 236-238
  lycopene 273-275
  Mediterranean Diet 215-216,
    219-220
  mustard seeds 260-261
  nuts 276
  Okinawa Diet 272
  olive oil 261-263
  omega-3 fatty acids 253-257
  onions 243-244
  Ornish program 217
  phytochemicals 235
  pomegranate 263-265
  portion control 241
  prostatitis and 84
  protein 240
  pumpkin seeds 265-267
  red meat 238-239
  rosemary 268-269
  salt 241
  saturated fat 236-239
  soy 269-271
  spinach 271-272
  supplements 281-330
  tomatoes 273-275
  trans fats 240
  water 278
  whole grains 277-278
Diethylstilbestrol (DES) 148
Digital rectal exam (DRE) 44, 102
Dihydrotestosterone (DHT)
  BPH and 39
  hair loss and 55
  hormone therapy and 145
  supplements and 322-330
Dill 268
Dipentum. See Olsalazine
Ditropan. See Oxybutynin
Docetaxel (Taxotere) 159
Doubling time 29, 87-88
Doxazosin (Cardura) 52, 56
Drugs. See Medications
Dry ejaculation 58
Dry orgasm 122
Duloxetin (Cymbalta) 77
Dutasteride (Avodart)
  for BPH 52, 53
  for prostate cancer 54

E

Edamame 269
Ellagic acid 264, 316-317
Epigallocatechin gallate (EGCG)
  258, 289
Epigenetics 90
Erectile dysfunction (ED). See
  Impotence
Exercise
  for prostatitis 80
  Ornish program 217

prostate health and 225-227
weight training 226
External beam radiation 130-132,
154, 166

F

Femara. *See* Letrozole
Finasteride (Proscar)
for BPH 52, 53
for hair loss 55
versus saw palmetto 328
Firmagon. *See* Degarelix
Fisetin 321
Fish
Mediterranean Diet and 219
omega-3 fatty acids in 253-257
Fish oil 297-299
flaxseed oil as alternative 324
Ornish program 217
Flaxseed oil 324-325
Flomax. *See* Tamsulosin
Flutamid 147
Folate 326
Folic acid 326
Foundation for Cancer Research
and Wellness 339

G

Gallic acid 301
Gamma-tocopherol 276, 308
Garlic 244. *See also* Aged garlic
extract (AGE)
Genetics
BPH and 39
prostate cancer and 89
Genistein 270, 318, 319
Gleason score 100-101
Glucosinolates 247-249, 260
Glycemic index 278-279

Glycyrrhizic acid 260
Gonadotropin-releasing hormone
(GnRH) agonists 146-147
Gonadotropin-releasing hormone
(GnRH) antagonists 147
Goserelin (Zoladex) 147
Grape seed extract (GSE) 301-302
Grapes 257-258
Green tea 258-259
Green tea extract 289-290
Grilling 239, 244-245, 268-269

H

Hair loss and BPH 55-56
Heart disease
controlling risk factors 221
impotence and 200
Mediterranean Diet and 219
PDE5 inhibitors and 204
prostate cancer and 220-221
Herbal remedies 268. *See also*
specific herbs
for BPH 51
for prostatitis 77
Heterocyclic amines (HCAs)
239, 268
HGPIN (high-grade prostatic
intraepithelial neoplasia) 98
High-grade prostatic intraep-
ithelial neoplasia (HGPIN) 98
High-intensity focused ultra-
sound (HIFU) 151-152, 154,
167
Hops 326-327
Hormone therapy 140-147
Hospitals 342-344
Hot flashes 306
Hytrin. *See* Terazosin

I

Ibuprofen
  for prostatitis 77
  PSA and 17
ILC (interstitial laser coagulation)
  68
Imipramine (Tofranil) 191
Impotence
  after biopsy 98-99
  after brachytherapy 135, 136,
    154
  after cryotherapy 154
  after external beam therapy
    154
  after HIFU 154
  after prostatectomy 117, 154,
    197
  age and 201
  alcohol and 199
  BPH medications and 52
  definition of 195
  depression and 200
  diabetes and 200
  heart disease and 200
  injury and 200
  medications and 201
  medications for 203-208
  nerve disorders and 200
  nerve-sparing prostatectomy
    and 122-124
  niacin for 200
  pomegranate for 264
  sleep test 210
  smoking and 199
  stress and 198-199
  support groups 338-339
  surgery for 209-210
  vacuum pump for 208-209
  weight and 201

Incontinence
  after brachytherapy 154
  after cryotherapy 154
  after external beam radiation
    154
  after HIFU 154
  after prostatectomy 118, 154
  artificial urinary sphincter for
    192-193
  biofeedback for 77-78, 189-190
  bladder pacemaker for 192
  bladder training and 188
  collagen injections for 191
  diet for 187-188
  Kegel exercises for 189
  male sling for 193
  medications for 191
  mixed incontinence 185
  overflow incontinence 185
  penile clamp for 191-192
  protective undergarments for
    187
  relaxation for 188-189
  stress incontinence 184
  support groups 337-338
  surgical complications 186
  urge incontinence 184
  visualization for 190
Inositol hexaniacinate 200
Insurance
  PDE5 inhibitors and 206
  vasodilators and 208
Intensity modulated radiation
  therapy (IMRT) 131
International Prostate Symptom
  Score (IPSS) 43-44
Interstitial laser coagulation
  (ILC) 68
Intravenous pyelography 46
Isothiocyanates 247

K

Kale 249
Kegel exercises
  BPH and 50-51
  incontinence and 189

L

Laparoscopic prostatectomy
  124-126, 169
Letrozole (Femara) 145
Leuprolide (Lupron) 147
Levitra. *See* Vardenafil
Libido. *See* Sex drive
Licorice 259-260
Lifestyle changes 218
Linolenic acid 248
Low-fat diet 236-238
Lupeol 305
Lupron. *See* Leuprolide
Luteinizing hormone-releasing
  hormone (LHRH) 145
Luteinizing hormone-releasing
  hormone (LHRH) agonists
  146-147
Luteinizing hormone-releasing
  hormone (LHRH) antagonists
  147
LUTS (lower urinary tract
  symptoms) 39-40
Lycopene 273-275, 293-296

M

Male menopause 142
Male sling 193
Male-pattern baldness and BPH
  55
Massage
  full-body 79
  prostate 79-80

Meares-Stamey four-cup test 82
Medications. *See also* specific
  medications
  androgen suppressants for
    BPH 53-54
  antihistamines and BPH 48
  aspirin 284-285
  BPH medications and erectile
    dysfunction 52
  chemotherapy 159
  decongestants and BPH 44, 48
  for impotence 203-208
  for incontinence 191
  for prostatitis 76, 84
  hormone therapy 140-147
  ibuprofen and PSA 16
  impotence and 201
  steroids for prostatitis 76
Mediterranean Diet 215-216,
  219-220
Melatonin 229
Mercury in fish 256
Mesalamine (Apriso) 194
Metastasis 236
Minipress. *See* Prazosin
Mint 268
Miso 270
MIST (minimally invasive surgi-
  cal technique) 63-65
Modified citrus pectin (MCP)
  300
Monounsaturated fat
  in olive oil 261-263
  Mediterranean Diet and 219,
    261-262
Multiple sclerosis 201
Muscadine 257, 297
Mustard greens 249
Mustard seeds 260-261
Myofascial trigger point therapy
  78

N

Natto 271
Nerve-sparing prostatectomy 122-124, 168
Neurogenic bladder 42
Niacin 200
Niaspan 200
Nicotinamide 200
Nicotinic acid 200
Niladron. *See* Nilutamide
Nilutamide (Niladron) 147
Nocturia 40
Nocturnal penile tumescence and rigidity (NPTR) test 210
Nomograms 151
Nonbacterial prostatitis. *See* Prostatitis
Nonsteroidal anti-inflammatory drugs (NSAIDs) 284
Nortriptyline (Aventyl) 77
Nutritional supplements. *See* Supplements
Nuts 277

O

Obesity. *See* Weight
Okinawa Diet 272
Oleic acid 262
Olive oil
    Mediterranean Diet and 219
    monounsaturated fat in 261-263
Olsalazine (Dipentum) 194
Omega-3 fatty acids
    in canola oil 248
    in fish 253-257, 299
    in fish oil supplements 297
    in flaxseed oil 324-325
    Mediterranean Diet and 219

Omega-6 fatty acids 298
Oncologist 14, 110
Onions 243-244
Orchiectomy 140
Oregano 268
Ornish program 216-217
Osteoporosis
    black cohosh for 306
    hormone therapy and 142
Overflow incontinence 185
Oxybutynin (Ditropan) 191
Oxytrol patch. *See* Oxybutynin

P

Pain management
    acupuncture 78-79
    massage 79
    myofascial trigger point therapy 78
    TENS 78
Papaverine (Pavabid) 207
Parkinson's disease 201
Parsley 268
Partin Tables 102-103
Pathological tumor grade 102
Pavabid. *See* Papaverine
PCA-3 urine test 105
PDE5 (phosphodiesterase type 5) inhibitors 203-206
Pectin 246, 300
Penile clamp 191-192
Penile implant 209-210
Peripheral zone of the prostate gland 35
Phentolamine (Regitine) 207
Phosphodiesterase type 5 inhibitors. *See* PDE5 (phosphodiesterase type 5) inhibitors

Photoselective vaporization of the prostate (PVP) 67
Phytochemicals 235
Polycyclic aromatic hydrocarbons (PAHs) 239, 245
Pomegranate 263-265
Portion control 241
Prazosin (Minipress) 56
Prednisone (Deltasone) 76
Premarin 148
Pressure-flow urodynamic study 46
Priapism 207
Proctitis 193-194
Proliferation 236
Propecia. See Finasteride
Proscar. See Finasteride
Prostate cancer
  abdominal fat and 223-224
  active surveillance and 111-115, 158
  age and 92
  alcohol and 227
  artificial light and 228
  biopsy for 95-99
  clinical trials 153
  diagnosis 88
  diet and 233-279
  dutasteride for 54
  exercise and 225-227
  growth rate 87, 93, 109-110
  heart disease and 220-221
  managing advanced disease 158-160
  medical treatments for 115-154
  Ornish program for 216-217
  prediction tool 151
  risk factors 89-90
  risk levels 99
  saturated fat and 237
  spread of 92-93
  stress and 230-231
  support groups 335-337
  symptoms 93-94
  testosterone and 91-92, 140-147
  tests for 104-106
  top-ranked hospitals for 342-344
  treatment comparison 154, 164
  tumor grading 102-104
  vasectomy and 91
  watchful waiting and 158
  weight and 221-222, 226
Prostate Cancer Foundation 340
Prostate Cancer Prevention Trial
  diet and BPH 234
  high-protein diet and LUTS 240
  lycopene and BPH 294
  red meat and prostate health 238
  vegetables and BPH 242
  vitamin D and prostate disease 286
  zinc and BPH 309
Prostate Cancer Research Institute 340
Prostate gland
  anatomy of 34-35
  illustrated 35
  signs of trouble 37
Prostate massage 79
Prostate stones 86
Prostate-specific antigen. See PSA (prostate-specific antigen)
Prostatectomy
  laparoscopic 124-126, 169
  nerve-sparing 122-124, 168
  overview 115-116
  radical 120-121, 167
  retropubic 62

Prostatectomy (*continued*)
  risks 117-119, 154
  robotic 126-129, 168
  suprapubic 62
  top-ranked hospitals for 342-
    344
Prostatitis
  abacterial 71
  acupuncture for 78-79
  acute bacterial 71, 82-83
  asymptomatic inflammatory 71
  bacterial 82-85
  biofeedback for 77-78
  Botox for 85
  caffeine and 84
  chronic bacterial 71, 83-84
  chronic nonbacterial 71-72
  constipation and 81
  cranberries for 252-253
  depression and 77
  diagnosing 81-82
  diet and 81, 84
  evaluating symptoms 72-75
  exercise for 80
  herbal remedies for 77
  massage for 79
  medications for 76, 84
  myofascial trigger point ther-
    apy for 78
  nonbacterial 71
  prostate massage for 79
  PSA and 16
  sexual intercourse for 85
  steroids for 76-77
  support groups 334-335
  surgery for 81
  symptoms 83, 84
  TENS for 78
  treatments 76-81
  TUMT for 81

Prostatitis Foundation 340
Protein 240
Proton beam radiation 133-134
Provenge. *See* Sipuleucel-T
PSA (prostate-specific antigen)
  after treatment 156-157
  age and 92
  bound 94
  definition of 10, 20, 101
  doubling time 29
  free 94
  measurement 22
  medications and 16
  race and 92
  saturated fat and 237
  sexual intercourse and 17
  stress and 230
PSA density 101
PSA test
  age and 26-27
  anxiety and 29-30
  baseline 29
  benefits of 16, 24, 30
  biopsy and 25, 94
  chronic disease and 27
  drawbacks of 14, 19, 21, 25, 31
  false negatives 25
  false positives 25, 29
  family history and 27
  frequency of 25
  insurance and 26
  interpreting results 28-30
  prostate cancer and 88
  race and 27
  screening guidelines 22-23,
    31-32
  side effects 30
PSA velocity 101-102
Pseudoephedrine (Chlor
  Trimeton) 191

Pumpkin seeds 265-267
PVP (photoselective vaporization of the prostate) 67-68
Pygeum 293

Q

Quercetin 287-288

R

Race
  BPH and 39
  prostate cancer and 89-90
  PSA levels and 92
  PSA test and 27
  vitamin D absorption and 286
Radiation therapy
  after prostatectomy 124
  brachytherapy 135-139
  external beam radiation 130-132
  impotence from 154
  incontinence from 154
  overview 129-130
  proctitis from 193-194
  proton beam radiation 133-134
  side effects 132
Radical prostatectomy 120-121, 167
Radionuclide scintigraphy 104-105
Raisins 267
Rapaflo. See Silodosin
Raspberries 247
Red clover 318
Regitine. See Phentolamine
Resistance training 226
Resveratrol 296-297
  in grapes 257-258
  Mediterranean Diet and 219

Resvinatrol 297
Retrograde ejaculation 58
Robotic prostatectomy 126-129, 168
Rosemary 268-269
Rye grass pollen extract 320-321

S

Salmon 256, 299
Salt 241
Saturated fat
  BPH and 234, 237
  prostate cancer and 234, 237
Saw palmetto 327-329
SELECT (Selenium and Vitamin E Cancer Prevention Trial) 315
Selenium 217, 314-315
Selenium and Vitamin E Cancer Prevention Trial (SELECT) 315
Seminal vesicle
  anatomy of 35
  prostate cancer and 93, 159
  prostatectomy and 121
Sepsis 99
Sex drive. See also Impotence
  hormone therapy and 143
Sexual intercourse
  for prostatitis 85
  PSA and 17
Sexually transmitted diseases 232
Sildenafil (Viagra) 203-206
Silodosin (Rapaflo) 56
Simon Foundation for Continence 341
Sipuleucel-T (Provenge) 159-160
Sitz bath 51, 85
Sleep
  prostate cancer and 228-230
  test for impotence 210

Slo-Niacin 200
Smoking
  beta carotene and 310
  BPH and 231
  impotence and 199
  prostate cancer and 231
  quitting 231-232
  vitamin E and 307
Soy 269-271, 319
Spectrographic endorectal mag-
  netic resonance imaging
  105-106
Spinach 271-272
Stents 69-70
Steroids 76-77
Stinging nettle extract 330
Strawberries 247
Stress
  active surveillance and 114
  BPH and 51
  impotence and 198-199
  Ornish program 217
  prostate cancer and 230-231
  reduction techniques 231
Stress incontinence 184
Sulfasalazine (Azulfidine) 194
Sulforaphane 247
Supplements
  African plum extract 292
  aged garlic extract (AGE) 316
  aspirin 284-285
  bee pollen extract 322-323
  beta carotene 310-311
  beta-sitosterol 302-303
  black cohosh 306-307
  black cumin seeds 303-304
  boron 267
  capsaicin 323-324
  conjugated linoleic acid
    (CLA) 312-314
  curcumin 290-292

ellagic acid 316-317
fisetin 321
fish oil 297-299
flaxseed oil 324-326
folic acid 326
genistein 319
grape seed extract (GSE) 301-
  302
green tea extract 289-290
guidelines 282-284
lupeol 305
lycopene 293-296
Ornish program 217
pectin 300
quercetin 287-288
red clover 318
resveratrol 296-297
rye grass pollen extract 320-321
saw palmetto 327-329
selenium 314-315
stinging nettle extract 330
testosterone and 322
vitamin C 311-312
vitamin D 285-287
vitamin E 307-308
xanthohumol 326-327
zinc 308-309
Surgery. See also Prostatectomy
  for impotence 209-210
  for prostate cancer 115-129,
    149-151
  for prostatitis 81
  hospital rankings 342-344
  impotence from 154, 197
  incontinence from 154, 186
  questions to ask 180-181
  second opinion 178-179
  surgical castration 140, 148-149
  versus brachytherapy 139
  weight and 224

T

Tadalafil (Cialis) 203

Tamsulosin (Flomax) 52, 56, 204, 328

Taxotere. *See* Docetaxel

Tempeh 270

TENS (transcutaneous electrical nerve stimulation) 78

Terazosin (Hytrin) 52, 56

Testosterone. *See also* Hormone therapy. *See also* Dihydrotestosterone (DHT)
  androgen deprivation therapy 140-147
  BPH and 38-39
  prostate cancer and 91-92
  supplements and 322-330
  surgical castration 148-149
  weight and 222

Texturized vegetable protein (TVP) 234

Thalidomide 163

The Prostate Net 341

Three-dimensional conformal radiation therapy (3D-CRT) 131

Thyme 268

Thymoquinone (TQ) 303

TNM (Tumor Node Metastases) system 103-104

Tofranil. *See* Imipramine

Tofu 234, 270

Tolterodine tartrate (Detrol) 191

Tomatoes 273-275, 294

Trans fats 240

Transcutaneous electrical nerve stimulation (TENS) 78

Transgenic adenocarcinoma of the mouse prostate (TRAMP) 320

Transition zone of the prostate gland 35

Transrectal ultrasonography (TRUS) 97

Transurethral electrovaporization (TUVP) 60-61

Transurethral incision of the prostate (TUIP) 62

Transurethral microwave thermotherapy (TUMT) 65-66, 81

Transurethral needle ablation (TUNA) 66-67

Transurethral resection of the prostate (TURP) 59-60, 158

Trelstar. *See* Triptorelin

Triptorelin (Trelstar) 147

TRUS (transrectal ultrasonography) 97

TUIP (transurethral incision of the prostate) 62

Tumor
  clinical grade 102
  Partin Tables 102-103
  pathological grade 102
  TNM cancer grading system 103

TUMT (transurethral microwave thermotherapy) 65-66, 81

TUNA (transurethral needle ablation) 66-67

Turmeric 290

TURP (transurethral resection of the prostate) 59-60, 158

TUVP (transurethral electrovaporization) 60-61

U

U.S. Preventive Services Task Force (USPSTF) 11

Ultrasound 45-46
Urethra 35
Urethral stricture 42, 118
Urethritis 185
Urge incontinence 184
Urinalysis 45, 82
Urinary incontinence. *See*
Incontinence
Urinary retention
acute 41
BPH and 41
Uroflowmetry 45
Urologist 14, 110, 173-175
Uroxatral. *See* Alfuzosin

V

Vacuum erection device (VED)
208-209
Vardenafil (Levitra) 203
Vasectomy 91
Vasodilators for impotence 206-
208
Viagra. *See* Sildenafil
Visualization 190
Vitamin C 311-312
in citrus fruits 251-252
Ornish program 217
supplemental and LUTS 252
Vitamin D 285-287
Vitamin E 307-308
in collard greens 249
in nuts 276
Ornish program 217
selenium and 314

W

Walnuts 276
Watchful waiting. *See also*
Active surveillance
BPH and 49
overview 169
prostate cancer and 158
Water 278
Water-induced thermotherapy
(WIT) 68-69
Watercress 249
Weather, effect on prostate 50
Weight
abdominal fat 223-224
body mass index (BMI) 222-
223
impotence and 201
prostate disease and 221-222
Weight training 226
Whole grains 277-278
WIT (water-induced ther-
motherapy) 68-69

X

Xanthohumol 326-327

Z

Zinc 308-309
Zoladex. *See* Goserelin
Zoledronic acid (Zometa) 145
Zometa. *See* Zoledronic acid